Parkinson's Disease

Questions and Answers

5TH EDITION

EDITOR/AUTHOR:

ROBERT A. HAUSER, MD
Professor of Neurology, Pharmacology and Experimental Therapeutics. Director, Parkinson's Disease and Movement Disorders Center, University of South Florida College of Medicine, Tampa General Healthcare, Tampa, FL

AUTHORS:

THERESA A. ZESIEWICZ, MD
Associate Professor of Neurology, Assistant Director, Parkinson's Disease and Movement Disorders Center, University of South Florida College of Medicine Tampa General Healthcare, Tampa, FL

KELLY E. LYONS, PhD
Research Associate Professor of Neurology, Director of Research and Education Parkinson's Disease and Movement Disorder Center, University of Kansas Medical Center, Kansas City, KS

RAJESH PAHWA, MD
Laverne and Joyce Rider Professor of Neurology, Director, Parkinson's Disease and Movement Disorder Center, University of Kansas Medical Center, Kansas City, KS

LAWRENCE GOLBE, MD
Professor of Neurology, University of Medicine and Dentistry of New Jersey Robert Wood Johnson Medical School, New Brunswick, NJ

MARK STACY, MD
Associate Professor of Neurology, Director, Duke University Movement Disorders Center, Duke University Medical Center, Durham, NC

WOLFGANG H. OERTEL, MD
Professor of Neurology, Philipps-University, Marburg, Germany

JEN C. MÖLLER, MD
Department of Neurology, Philipps-University, Marburg, Germany

WERNER POEWE, MD
Professor of Neurology, Medical University, Innsbruck, Austria

ELISABETH WOLF, MD
Dept. of Neurology, Medical University, Innsbruck, Austria

PUBLISHING
INTERNATIONAL

Cover Design and Artwork by:

SMK Design

merit
PUBLISHING
INTERNATIONAL

Parkinson's Disease

Questions and Answers

5TH EDITION

MERIT PUBLISHING INTERNATIONAL

European address:
50 Highpoint, Heath Road
Weybridge, Surrey KT13 8TP
England

Tel: (44) (0) 1932 844526
Fax: (44) (0) 1932 820419

North American address:
5840 Corporate Way, Suite 200
West Palm Beach, FL 33407
USA

Tel: 561 697 1116
Fax: 561 477 4961

Web: www.meritpublishing.com

ISBN: 1 873413 63 7
978 1 873413 63 0

merit
PUBLISHING
INTERNATIONAL

Parkinson's Disease

CONTENTS

Parkinson's Disease

Parkinson's Disease

Disease

Questions and Answers

5TH EDITION

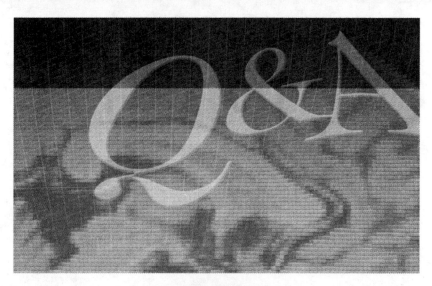

EDITOR/AUTHOR:

ROBERT A. HAUSER

AUTHORS:

THERESA A. ZESIEWICZ, KELLY E. LYONS, RAJESH PAHWA, LAWRENCE GOLBE, MARK STACY
WOLFGANG H. OERTEL, JEN C. MÖLLER, WERNER POEWE, ELISABETH WOLF

merit
PUBLISHING
INTERNATIONAL

Parkinson's Disease

CHAPTER 1

INTRODUCTION TO PARKINSON'S DISEASE

Theresa A. Zesiewicz, Robert A. Hauser

Parkinson's disease is a progressive, neurologic disorder caused by a degeneration of dopamine neurons. James Parkinson first described the disease in 1817[1]. Since then, tremendous advances have been made in understanding its pathophysiology and in developing effective treatments. The landmark discovery that levodopa ameliorates symptoms came in the late 1960s. Even today, Parkinson's disease remains one of the few neurodegenerative diseases whose symptoms can be improved with medication therapy. Exciting research into emerging medical and surgical treatments continues at a breathtaking pace. New clues as to its cause are now emerging. This chapter introduces Parkinson's disease, its history, and current concepts of pathophysiology.

What causes the symptoms of Parkinson's disease?

Movement of the body is initiated in an area of the brain called the motor cortex. The main motor pathway consists of the pyramidal system, which extends from the motor cortex to the spinal cord. Lower motor neurons carry signals from the spinal cord to muscles to produce movement. The pyramidal system is modulated by the "extrapyramidal" circuit, which includes the substantia nigra, striatum, subthalamic nucleus, the external and internal segments of the globus pallidus, and the thalamus. The extrapyramidal system can either promote or inhibit movement depending on tonic dopamine innervation of the striatum. Normal movement is dependent on appropriate dopamine production by substantia nigra neurons innervating the striatum (figure 1.1).

Parkinson's disease is associated with a massive degeneration of dopaminergic nigrostriatal neurons. When approximately sixty to eighty percent of the dopamine-producing neurons of the substantia nigra are lost, the extrapyramidal system is no longer able to effectively promote movement, and the symptoms of Parkinson's disease appear.

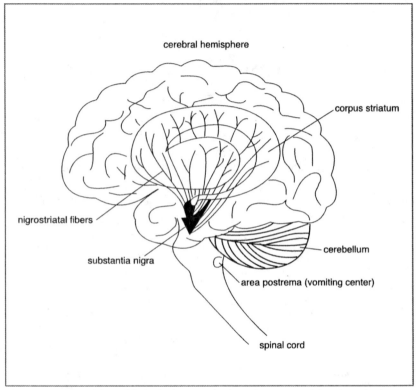

Figure 1.1. *Lateral view of the brain demonstrates dopamine neurons of the substantia nigra innervating the striatum.*

Pathological studies indicate that the disease can be divided into six stages. Stages one and two are "presymptomatic" and characterized by inclusion bodies in the medulla oblongata, pontine tegmentum, olfactory bulb and anterior olfactory nucleus. Dysfunction in these areas may cause loss of smell and sleep abnormalities. Stages three and four comprise the "symptomatic phases" when the substantia nigra and other areas of the midbrain and forebrain undergo degeneration, and patients show the classic signs of Parkinson's disease. In stages five and six, the neocortex is affected, and patients may experience dementia (Figure 1.2) [2].

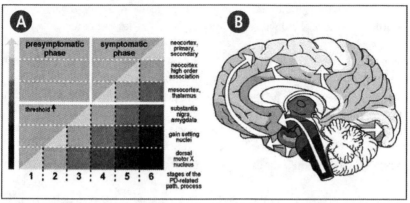

Figure 1.2. *PD presymptomatic and symptomatic phases.* **A** *The presymptomatic phase is marked by the appearance of Lewy neurites/bodies in the brains of asymptomatic persons. In the symptomatic phase, the individual neuropathological threshold is exceeded (black arrow). The increasing slope and intensity of the shaded areas below the diagonal indicate the growing severity of the pathology in vulnerable brain regions (right). The severity of the pathology is indicated by darker degrees of shading.* **B** *Diagram showing the ascending pathological process (white arrows). The shading intensity of the colored areas corresponds to that in* **A**

Cell and tissue Research, 318 No.1, 2004, 121-134, Braak H, Ghebremedhin E, Rub U, Bratzke H, Del Tredici K, Figure A1 and B1.
With kind permission of Springer Science and Business media.

What are the clinical features of Parkinson's disease?

Four main motor features characterize Parkinson's disease:

- resting tremor (shaking back and forth when the limb is relaxed)

- bradykinesia (slowness of movement)

- rigidity (stiffness, or resistance of the limb to passive movement when the limb is relaxed)

- postural instability (poor balance)

Onset of symptoms is asymmetric with one limb, usually an arm, affected first. Signs and symptoms then spread to the other limb on that side and later affect the limbs of the opposite side. Resting tremor, bradykinesia, and rigidity are relatively early signs often apparent in the first-affected extremity. Postural instability, or imbalance, is a late symptom typically emerging ten or more years into the disease.

Other common signs include shuffling gait, stooped posture, difficulty with fine coordinated movements, and micrographia (small handwriting). Non-motor symptoms of the disease include sleep disorders, fatigue, sexual dysfunction, sensory symptoms, autonomic dysfunction, cognitive abnormalities, and mood disorders. These will be discussed in greater detail in a later chapter.

In one study, patients reported tremor to be the most troublesome aspect of PD during the first decade following diagnosis. Imbalance was the chief complaint of patients 12-14 years after diagnosis[3]. However, several recent studies indicate that the non-motor symptoms of the disease may be as troublesome as motor symptoms[4].

How did Parkinson's disease get its name?

James Parkinson, a 19th century English physician, was the first to publish an accurate description of the disease in a pamphlet entitled, "An Essay on the Shaking Palsy"[1]. He had encountered several patients who exhibited resting tremor, stooped posture, shuffling gait, and retropulsion (falling backward). He recognized that symptoms progressively worsened, ultimately leading to death from complications due to immobility. The tremor was present with the limbs at rest. He dubbed the disease "paralysis agitans", paralysis referring to the paucity of movement and agitans referring to the tremor.

Although Parkinson did not identify abnormalities in muscle tone or cognition in his patients, the bulk of his description of the disease was remarkably accurate. The French physician Jean Marie Charcot added muscular rigidity, micrographia, sensory changes, and several other features to Parkinson's original description, and named it after the physician who first clearly described it[5].

Who gets Parkinson's disease?

Parkinson's disease commonly occurs in older individuals, although it may also occur in young adults. It is present worldwide and in all populations[6]. Men have a slightly higher prevalence rate than women[7]. No race or specific region of the world has been found to be completely devoid of the disease.

What is the mean age of onset of Parkinson's disease?

The mean age of onset of Parkinson's disease is approximately 60 years. It usually occurs in patients over 50 years of age, and onset before age 25 is rare. The incidence and prevalence of the disease generally increase with increasing age[7]. Age-specific death rates for Parkinson's disease increased in the elderly in the United States from 1962 through 1984, and decreased in younger age groups[8]. The decreased mortality in younger individuals is likely the result of the introduction of dopamine replacement medical therapy.

How common is Parkinson's disease?

"Prevalence" and "incidence" are two terms used to describe the frequency of a disease. Prevalence refers to the total number of people with the disease in a population at a given time. Incidence is the number of new cases of the disease diagnosed in a population during a given time period.

The prevalence of Parkinson's disease (PD) increases with age. Average crude prevalence rates for Parkinson's disease have been estimated at 120-180 per 100,000 in Caucasian populations[6] and the prevalence of the disease in individuals over 65 years of age is roughly 1%. By the eighth decade, the prevalence of PD in North America and Europe is estimated to be 2-3%[9]. Studies conducted over the last century in Rochester, Minnesota have not uncovered a change in the prevalence of Parkinson's disease in the last fifty years[10]. Incidence rates have been estimated at 20 per 100,000. The lifetime risk of developing PD may be as high as 1 in 40[11].

Does Parkinson's disease occur more frequently in certain locations?

North America and Europe have fairly high prevalence rates of PD while the lowest prevalence rates have been found in China, Nigeria, and Sardinia[6]. The Parsi community of Bombay, India was found to have a high prevalence rate[12]. The Parsis migrated to India between the seventh and tenth centuries from Iran. They have a closed community and rarely allow intermarriages with other races or religious groups. A recent study found that Sydney, Australia has one of the highest prevalence rates of PD in a developed country[13]. Combining data from two Sydney studies revealed that the prevalence rate is 780/100,000. A high prevalence rate for PD was also reported in Argentina and Sicily[14]. Age-adjusted prevalence rates in Sicily and Junin, a Buenos Aires province in Argentina, were approximately 206/100,000[14,15,12]. Whether genetic factors in a closed community or some environmental toxin present in the area is causing this high prevalence is unknown.

Is Parkinson's disease more common in Caucasians or African-Americans?

Studies conducted in the United States have generally found a lower prevalence of Parkinson's disease among African-Americans[16]. Even in Africa, the prevalence has been found to be lower in blacks than in whites or Indians[17]. However, in a door-to-door survey conducted in Copiah County, Mississippi, prevalence among blacks was similar to that among whites when relatively loose diagnostic criteria were employed[18]. When more rigid diagnostic criteria were used, whites continued to have a higher prevalence.

Mayeux et al. estimated the prevalence and incidence of PD over a four-year period in a culturally diverse community in New York City, and found a prevalence rate of 107 per 100,000 and an incidence rate of 13 per 100,000 person-years. Age-adjusted prevalence rates were lower for blacks than for whites and Hispanics. However, the age-adjusted incidence rate was highest for black men (black men over age 75 had the highest incidence rate among all groups). A higher mortality rate or delay in diagnosis among black men may account for these findings[19]. Further studies are needed to substantiate the belief that Parkinson's disease is more common in Caucasians and to determine whether access to healthcare or other factors differentially affect the incidence and prevalence of PD in various populations.

What factors are associated with the development of Parkinson's disease?

There is interest in whether exposure to a toxin or multiple toxins might cause Parkinson's disease. It may not be coincidence that James Parkinson's original description of the disease in 1817 occurred at the beginning of the industrial revolution in the United States[20]. Several associations between environmental exposures and Parkinson's disease have been identified including rural living, well-water intake, vegetable farming, exposure to wood pulp, and exposure to pesticides[6].

Some of these associations are controversial and no environmental toxin has been identified that might be causative for most patients with Parkinson's disease. Nonetheless, interest in environmental toxins was greatly bolstered by the discovery that MPTP, a heroin derivative, caused a Parkinson's disease-like illness in young adults who injected themselves with this contaminant[21]. Animals made parkinsonian through injection of MPTP provide a valuable research tool.

Are any occupations associated with the development of Parkinson's disease?

One study that used a medical records-linkage system to identify subjects who developed PD in Olmsted County, MN, from 1976 through 1995 found that patients with nine or more years of education were at increased risk of PD (OR = 2.0; 95% CI = 1.1 to 3.6; p = 0.02) [22]. Physicians were also at significantly increased risk for PD.

What is the prognosis of Parkinson's disease?

Parkinson's disease is a chronic, degenerative disease that usually progresses fairly slowly. Although an average rate of progression can be defined, it is not possible to accurately predict prognosis for an individual patient. Most patients initially do very well on medication for four to six years. Between five and ten years most patients experience medication-related difficulty and many develop poor balance by ten to twelve years. It takes an average of two and a half years to progress from stage to stage (see chapter 4), although this is only a rough guideline [23].

Before the introduction of levodopa, Parkinson's disease dramatically reduced life expectancy. The mortality rate for Parkinson's disease patients was almost three times that of the general population. Treatment with dopamine replacement therapy essentially normalized life expectancy and death rates for Parkinson's disease and non-Parkinson's individuals are now approximately equal [23]. A study conducted in Olmsted County, Minnesota found that patients diagnosed with PD before age 60 had a comparable relative survival rate to the general population, while patients diagnosed at an older age had a lower relative survival rate than expected [24].

Risk factors for more rapid progression of disability include older age at onset [25], lack of tremor [26], and rigidity or bradykinesia as presenting features [26]. Risk factors for nursing home placement include dementia and older age at disease onset [27].

What is the basic anatomy and pharmacology of Parkinson's disease?

The classic signs of Parkinson's disease are due to abnormalities in the extrapyramidal motor circuit. The basal ganglia are subcortical nuclei comprised of three components: the caudate nucleus, the putamen and the globus pallidus (figure 1.3). The caudate nucleus consists of a "head" which lies next to the lateral ventricle, the "body" which lies lateral to the thalamus, and the "tail" which enters the temporal lobe. The putamen and globus pallidus lie between the internal and external capsules, with the putamen situated laterally. The globus pallidus is composed of medial and lateral segments.

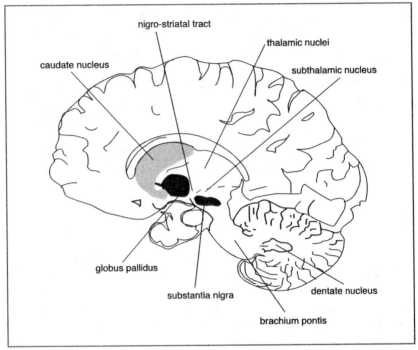

Figure 1.3. *Lateral view of the brain indicating positions of the substantia nigra, caudate, subthalamic nucleus and thalamus.*

Also involved in the extrapyramidal circuit is the substantia nigra. This structure is located in the midbrain, ventral to the tegmentum. It is composed of a pigment-rich area called the "zona compacta" and a relatively cell-poor region called the "zona reticulata". Neurons in the zona compacta are responsible for the production of dopamine, while the zona reticulata primarily produces GABA (gamma-amino-butyric acid).

The ability to produce movement is dependent on a complex motor circuit involving the substantia nigra, basal ganglia, subthalamic nucleus, thalamus, and the cerebral cortex (figure 1.4). Signals from the cerebral cortex are processed through the motor circuit and returned to the same areas by a feedback pathway [28]. The output from the motor circuit is directed through the internal segment of the globus pallidus (GPi) and the substantia nigra pars reticulata (SNr). This inhibitory output is directed to the thalamocortical pathway and suppresses movement.

There are two pathways within the extrapyramidal system: a direct and an indirect pathway. In the direct pathway, outflow from the striatum (putamen and caudate) inhibits the GPi and SNr. The indirect pathway contains inhibitory connections between 1) the striatum and the external segment of the globus pallidus (GPe), and 2) the globus pallidus externa (GPe) and the subthalamic nucleus (STN). The subthalamic nucleus has an excitatory influence on the GPi and SNr. The GPi/SNr sends inhibitory efferents to the ventral lateral (VL) nucleus of the thalamus. Putamenal neurons containing D1 receptors comprise the direct pathway and project to the GPi. Putamenal neurons containing D2 receptors are part of the indirect pathway and project to the GPe. Dopamine activates the direct pathway and inhibits the indirect pathway.

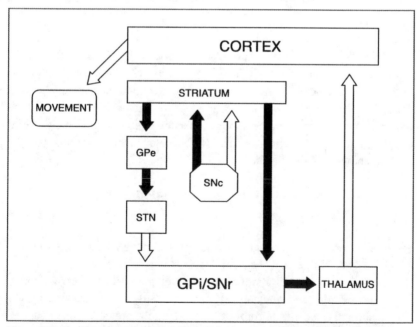

Figure 1.4. *Schematic representation of the normal motor circuit demonstrating the direct and indirect pathways. See text for details. Black arrows represent inhibition and white arrows represent stimulation. SNc = substantia nigra pars compacta; GPe = globus pallidus externa; STN = subthalamic nucleus; GPi = globus pallidus interna; SNr = substantia nigra pars reticulata.*

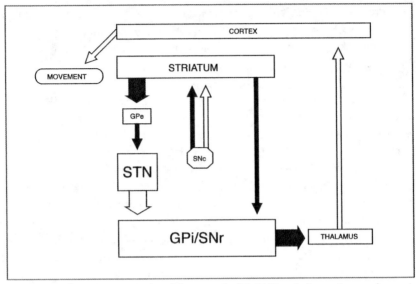

Figure 1.5. *Schematic representation of the motor circuit in Parkinson's disease. Decreased dopamine production by the SNc leads to overinhibition of the thalamocortical pathway. See text for details.*

In Parkinson's disease, decreased production of dopamine by the SNc leads to increased inhibitory output from the GPi/SNr (figure 1.5). This increased inhibition of the thalamocortical pathway suppresses movement. Via the direct pathway, low dopamine levels decrease inhibition of the GPi/SNr, causing overinhibition of the thalamus. Via the indirect pathway, low dopamine levels increase inhibition of the GPe, resulting in "disinhibition" of the STN. Increased STN output promotes GPi/SNr inhibition of the thalamus.

What histopathologic features are associated with Parkinson's disease?

Parkinson's disease involves a degeneration of cells in the substantia nigra pars compacta. The lightly melanized ventral layer in the pars compacta is primarily affected [29]. Clinical manifestations occur when roughly 60% of neurons in this region are lost. Motor symptomatology generally reflects advancing neuronal loss in the substantia nigra [29-32]. In contrast to PD where the greatest loss of neurons is in the ventral layer, with aging there is a greater loss of neurons in the dorsal tier.

It is estimated that with advancing age, 2.1% of neurons in the ventral tier are lost per decade, while 6.9% of neurons degenerate in the dorsal tier [31]. Cell loss in PD is not confined solely to the substantia nigra but also affects the locus ceruleus, thalamus, cerebral cortex, and autonomic nervous system. Neurotransmitter abnormalities involve the adrenergic, cholinergic and serotonergic as well as the dopaminergic system.

The pathological determination of Parkinson's disease includes the identification of Lewy bodies [29]. These are eosinophilic, concentric, hyaline inclusions present in the cytoplasm of some remaining substantia nigra pars compacta neurons. They can also be found in the locus ceruleus, autonomic neurons, and other areas. Lewy bodies consist of a dense center and a pale staining, peripheral halo. The outer layer consists of cytoskeletal elements.

It was recently discovered that alpha-synuclein is a major structural component of Lewy bodies [33]. This is an important observation because abnormalities in the gene for alpha-synuclein cause PD in some families (see chapter 2). Lewy bodies have also been found in other degenerative disorders and in some elderly individuals without parkinsonian features. The presence of Lewy bodies at autopsy in some "normal" individuals may suggest that they had preclinical Parkinson's disease, and would have developed signs and symptoms if they had lived longer. Incidental Lewy bodies are present in about 1% of the non-parkinsonian population dying at 50-59 years of age [34,35].

The prevalence of incidental Lewy bodies rises to 10% for individuals dying at 80-89 years of age. This compares with a 1-2% prevalence of PD in the 80-89-year-old age group, suggesting that Lewy bodies are present during a preclinical period before symptoms become apparent [34,35]. Neurodegenerative diseases marked by Lewy bodies include corticobasal degeneration, motor neuron disease, ataxia telangiectasia, subacute sclerosing panencephalitis, and Hallevorden Spatz disease [34].

What is the neurochemistry of Parkinson's disease?

Dopamine and other cathecholamines are synthesized from tyrosine by the following pathway:

tyrosine -> 3,4-dihydroxyphenylalanine (DOPA) -> dopamine -> norepinephrine -> epinephrine.

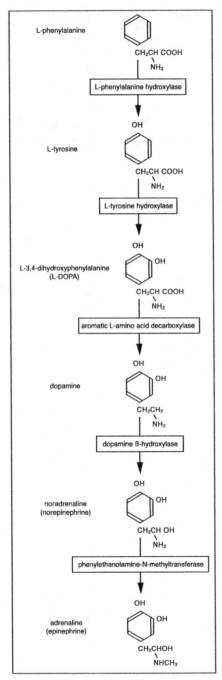

The rate-limiting step in the formation of dopamine is the hydroxylation of tyrosine to form DOPA. This step is catalyzed by the protein tyrosine hydroxylase (figure 1.6). Tyrosine hydroxylase is a marker of dopamine neurons. It is decreased in the substantia nigra of Parkinson's disease patients. Dopamine and its metabolites, homovanillic acid (HVA) and dihydroxyphenylacetic acid (DOPAC), are reduced in the striatum, the primary target of dopamine neurons [36]. Dopamine loss is more extensive in the putamen than in the caudate [37]. Dopamine levels are also reduced in the hypothalamus, mesolimbic, and mesocortical areas.

Once formed, two enzymes metabolize dopamine-monoamine oxidase (MAO), which deaminates dopamine intraneuronally, and catechol-O-methyl transferase (COMT), which methylates dopamine outside the neuron [38] (figure 1.7). MAO exists in two forms: MAO-A and MAO-B. MAO-B is the predominant form in the brain and is found on the outer membrane of mitochondria. MAO-B inhibitors increase levels of striatal dopamine. COMT methylates dopamine extraneuronally by catalyzing the transfer of a methyl group from S-adenosyl-L-methionine to the m-hydroxy group of dopamine. Dopamine is also deactivated by neuronal reuptake via the dopamine transporter.

Figure 1.6. *Synthesis of dopamine and other catecholamines.*

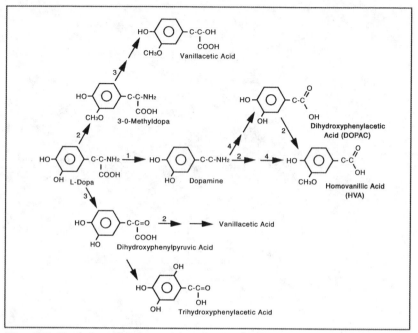

Figure 1.7. *Metabolism of levodopa and dopamine. 1=aromatic amino acid decarboxylase; 2=catechol-O-methyltransferase; 3=tyrosine aminotransferase; 4=monoamine oxidase.*

What are the different types of dopamine receptors?

Receptors are macromolecules composed of proteins located on neuronal membranes (figure 1.8). The two main types of dopamine receptors are D1 and D2 [39,40] Dopamine functions by modulating the direct and indirect pathways of the extrapyramidal motor circuit through its effect on D1 and D2 receptors. Dopamine receptors are linked to a guanine nucleotide-binding protein (G-protein), to form a complex, which interacts with adenyl cyclase to control formation of the second messenger, adenylate cyclase (figure 1.9). The D1 receptor family includes D1 and D5 receptors, while D2 includes D2, D3, and D4 receptors (figure 1.10). Receptors in the D1 family increase cyclic AMP, while those in the D2 family reduce cyclic AMP [39-41]. D2 receptor activation is important in the anti-parkinsonian response to dopamine agonist medications. The role of D1 receptor activation in the response to medications is less clear.

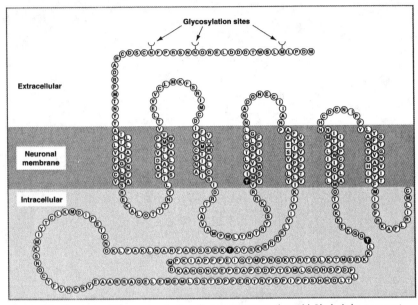

Figure 1.8. *Structure of D2 receptor. Each circle represents an amino acid. Black circles represent phosphorylation sites.*

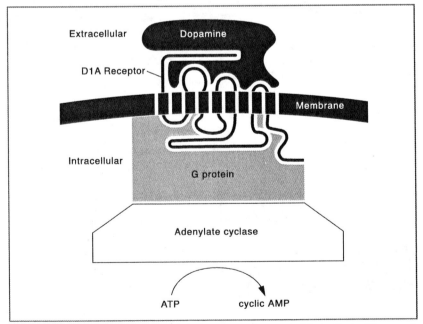

Figure 1.9. *D1 receptor. The receptor is linked to a G protein to control the synthesis of the second messsenger, cyclic AMP.*

	D1		D2		
Currently used term	A	B	A	B	C
Previously used term	D1	D5	D2	D3	D4
Location (high concentrations)	Striatum Nucleus accumbens Amygdala Olfactory bulb	Hippocampus Hypothalamus	Striatum Nucleus accumbens Substantia nigra Olfactory bulb	Hypothalamus Nucleus accumbens Olfactory bulb	Frontal cortex Midbrain Medulla
Action (information is limited to biochemical indexes)	Increases cyclic AMP	Increases cyclic AMP	Reduces cyclic AMP Opens potassium channels Closes calcium channels	Reduces cyclic AMP	Reduces cyclic AMP

Figure 1.10. *Distribution and function of dopamine receptors.*

Are there tests available to diagnose Parkinson's disease?

The diagnosis of Parkinson's disease is made by clinical evaluation and there are currently no simple, widely available laboratory tests that make the diagnosis. Fluorodopa positron emission tomography (PET) is a useful index of striatal dopaminergic function [42] but is expensive and not widely available. Single photon emission computerized tomography (SPECT) using radioisotopes that bind to the dopamine transporter on nigrostriatal neuron terminals is also emerging as a useful modality [43]. Further development of SPECT technology may provide a widely available and relatively inexpensive diagnostic tool in the near future.

Parkinson's Disease

CHAPTER 2

ETIOLOGY OF PARKINSON'S DISEASE

Lawrence I. Golbe

Although the cause of Parkinson's disease is unknown, the modern consensus is that most cases of PD are the product of a combination of genetic and environmental factors. Under this "multifactorial" hypothesis, PD in any individual is the result of several factors and the precise combination of causes varies across individuals. This could explain how a disorder with a prominent genetic component occurs in a sporadic fashion in a majority of cases. Similarly, the multifactorial hypothesis could explain how a disorder with a major exogenous toxic component displays no clear geographical or occupational predilection.

To what extent is Parkinson's disease an inherited disorder?

About 20% of people with PD know of an affected first-degree relative. For individuals without PD, the figure is about 5% [1]. The ratio of these figures, a measure of familial aggregation, is lower than that of well-recognized adult-onset genetic disorders such as Huntington's disease. While the risk of developing PD some time during life is approximately 2% for the general population, it rises to 5-6% for those with a parent with PD and to 20-25% for those with both a parent and a sibling with PD [2]. But these data merely show that PD clusters within families.

A powerful method to examine the genetic component of a disease is to study twins with regard to "concordance," the fraction of twin pairs that both have the disease. For a disease caused by a single genetic abnormality that is fully penetrant (i.e., where all carriers of the disease gene develop the disease), all monozygotic (MZ) twin pairs but only half of dizygotic (DZ) twin pairs will be concordant.

MZ, or identical twins, come from division of a single egg and sperm union and therefore have identical sets of genes. DZ, or fraternal twins, come from two different egg and sperm unions, like siblings, and share approximately 50% of genes. For a fully penetrant disease gene, if one MZ twin has the disease, the other will, too (concordance of 1 or 100%). For DZ pairs, if one twin has the disease, the other has a 50% chance of having it too concordance of .5 or 50%). Thus, the MZ:DZ concordance ratio would be 2:1.

For genetic traits that, like most, are less than fully penetrant, the MZ:DZ concordance ratio remains 2:1 as expression of the disease is proportionally decreased in all individuals. For example if 50% of MZ twin pairs were concordant and 25% of DZ twin pairs were concordant, the MZ:DZ concordance ratio would be 2:1 and one could conclude that the disease was caused by a genetic abnormality that is expressed in 50% of individuals who have it. For a disease that is due entirely to an environmental cause, the MZ:DZ concordance ratio would be 1:1 because genetic status would be irrelevant. Thus, the higher the MZ:DZ concordance ratio, the greater the likelihood of a genetic cause for a disease, and the lower the MZ:DZ ratio the greater the likelihood of an environmental cause.

What is the twin concordance ratio for PD?

Twin studies that rely on clinical examination to determine the presence or absence of PD, if taken at face value, generate low MZ:DZ concordance ratios, suggesting at most a weak genetic influence or one that occurs only for younger-onset cases [3,4]. However, a study that used the far more sensitive method of positron emission tomographic (PET) imaging of dopamine neurons using (18F)-DOPA found that 55% of MZ pairs but only 18% of DZ pairs are concordant, a result strongly suggestive of a genetic cause. When the scans were repeated an average of four years later in order to measure rate of decline of dopaminergic function, the results were even more strongly supportive of a genetic cause, with MZ:DZ concordances of 75% and 22% [5].

MZ:DZ concordance ratios, like these, that are above 2:1, suggest that more than one gene abnormality is required to cause the disease in an individual. This is because if two or three gene abnormalities are required to cause the disease (and are fully penetrant), all MZ pairs would be concordant but fewer than 50% of DZ pairs would be concordant.

The issue of genetic contribution to apparently sporadic PD was examined in a very different way by researchers in Iceland, where centuries of genealogical records document distant familial relationships among most of the living population [6]. They randomly chose a number of patients with sporadic PD and a similar number of controls. They then randomly formed pairs of patients and pairs of controls and examined the genealogical records to quantify the closeness of the relationship within each pair. The relationships proved to be much closer for the patients than for the controls, suggesting that PD, at least in Iceland, tends to be hereditary, but with low penetrance that creates an appearance of sporadic occurrence.

Are there families in whom Parkinson's disease is clearly inherited?

One large family with highly penetrant, autosomal dominant, autopsy proven PD, originated in the town of Contursi in the Salerno province of southern Italy[7] and has been dubbed the "Contursi kindred." Its 60 affected individuals were characterized by early age of disease onset (mean age of 47.5 years), rapid progression (death at a mean age of 56.1 years), paucity of tremor and a good response to levodopa therapy. A few had cortical dementia that is quite unusual for PD, but for the most part, the range of clinical pictures was similar to that of sporadic PD. Linkage analysis incriminated a region in chromosome 4q21-23[8]. Sequencing of several candidate genes in that region revealed an A for G substitution at base 209 of the alpha-synuclein gene[9]. This was considered a candidate only because a fragment of the alpha-synuclein protein was known to occur in amyloid plaques of Alzheimer's disease. The single base-pair missense mutation codes for a substitution of threonine for alanine at amino acid 53 (A53T).

After the discovery of the A53T mutation in the Contursi kindred, geneticists were able to test specifically for that mutation and others in the alpha-synuclein gene in patients with sporadic PD or with familial PD where the family was too small for linkage analysis on its own. In this way, the A53T mutation was found in 12 small families, all of Greek origin[10]. A German family was found to have a different point mutation in the alpha-synuclein gene (a substitution of C for G at base 88, producing a substitution of proline for alanine at amino acid 30)[11]. A Spanish family with PD has a lys for glu mutation at amino acid 46[12]. An extended American family of northern European background (the Iowa kindred) has, in chromosome four of affected individuals, two extra copies of the region that includes the alpha-synuclein gene[13]. A French family has one extra copy[14]. The alpha-synuclein mutations causing PD are together termed "PARK1."

What does alpha-synuclein do?

Alpha-synuclein is a protein found abundantly at presynaptic nerve terminals in normal brain, particularly in the olfactory bulb and tract, hypothalamus, and substantia nigra. It is involved in maintenance and intracellular transport of dopamine vesicles before they release their contents into the synapse [15]. PARK1 mutations involving point mutations disrupt the alpha-helical portion of the alpha-synuclein molecule, substituting a beta sheet configuration. This appears to produce abnormal aggregation of alpha-synuclein [9]. The triplication or duplication mutations probably act by overproducing alpha-synuclein, causing it to aggregate via excessive concentration.

The mechanism by which alpha-synuclein aggregation leads to cell death is still being worked out. It may be related to the ability of an early stage of such aggregates ("protoaggregates" or "oligomers") to create pores in plasma membranes [16]. Perhaps the most important such membrane undergoing this sort of damage is that of the mitochondria. This not only degrades the cell's energy production but also allows leakage of certain mitochondrial contents that activate the cell's apoptotic pathway, setting in motion a process toward cell death. Another hypothesis is that the misfolded or overabundant alpha-synuclein clogs or overwhelms the proteasome system, which has primary responsibility for degrading excessive, defective or worn-out proteins. This may allow all manner of potentially toxic protein fragments to cause damage of various sorts. Quite likely the answer is a combination of these mechanisms.

Are abnormalities of alpha-synuclein found in non-familial Parkinson's disease?

Within days after the 1997 publication of the mutation causing PD in the Contursi kindred, several labs applied anti-alpha-synuclein immunostains to PD brains, revealing that alpha-synuclein is a major component of Lewy bodies, the histopathologic hallmark of PD [17]. This demonstrates that abnormal aggregation of alpha-synuclein occurs in all PD. It suggests that alpha-synuclein is probably an important component in the cascade of events leading to neuronal death in PD even though alpha-synuclein mutations are absent in sporadic PD and most familial PD.

The role of alpha-synuclein in sporadic PD has become a major line of inquiry for neuroscientists. Insertion of abnormal alpha-synuclein genes has allowed development of PD models in the mouse, fruit fly and roundworm [18].

Some important discoveries:

Dopamine itself promotes alpha-synuclein aggregation [19,20] and mutant alpha-synuclein is most deleterious in dopaminergic neurons. This could explain the predilection of the PD disease process for dopamine neurons.

Genetically engineered absence of alpha-synuclein protects against the mitochondrial damage caused by MPTP, an important dopamine-neuron-related toxin that will be discussed below [21]. This suggests that alpha-synuclein is an indispensable participant in that toxic process.

Certain commonly used pesticides [22] and metals [23] promote alpha-synuclein aggregation, perhaps explaining the epidemiologic association of PD with those exposures.

Heat-shock proteins interfere with alpha-synuclein aggregation and its toxicity [24] and geldanamycin, an inducer of heat-shock protein, prevents the neuronal degeneration completely [25]. Such insights could easily lead to preventions for PD.

Abnormal aggregation of tau protein, which accumulates in Alzheimer's disease and about a dozen other neurodegenerative disorders, occurs to a degree in PD, where it may stimulate the aggregation of alpha-synuclein, and vice versa [26,27].

What other unusual PD-causing genes have shed light on the etiology of all PD?

PARK2 or parkin is a gene that when mutated causes autosomal recessive juvenile parkinsonism (AR-JP) [28]. The gene was originally found in Japanese families [29] but has since been found in many other populations [30]. AR-JP is characterized by early onset parkinsonism (before age 40 and often before 30), slow disease progression, improvement following sleep, good response to levodopa therapy and levodopa-induced dyskinesias [28], without dementia or autonomic symptoms. Pathologically, there is marked neuronal loss in the substantia nigra and locus ceruleus, without Lewy bodies.

The gene is at chromosome 6 (6q25.2-q27). A huge range of mutations in the large parkin gene has been described, from large deletions to single base substitutions. AR-JP caused by parkin mutations ordinarily requires that both copies of chromosome 6 carry the same mutation (homozygosity) or that each copy carry a different mutation (duplex heterozygosity). But individuals with only one copy of a small parkin mutation (heterozygosity) can have late-life onset of symptoms and receive a diagnosis of idiopathic PD [31].

In a typical clinical series, in 307 families with familial PD, 16 (5%) harbored a parkin mutation [32]. Of the early-onset families, 18% carried a mutation and of the late-onset families, 2% did so. In 10 families, all of the affected individuals were heterozygotes.

Parkin protein is a ubiquitin ligase, an enzyme that cuts the polyubiquitin chain as part of the process that delivers defective or worn-out proteins to the proteasome for disposal and recycling of their component amino acids[33]. Parkin dysfunction therefore permits accumulation of an as-yet unidentified waste protein, which presumably aggregates to produce neuronal loss. There is mounting evidence that sporadic PD involves dysfunction of the ubiquitin-proteasome system[34], possibly via impaired breakdown of alpha-synuclein[35]. Better understanding of this role could soon offer excellent opportunities for pharmacologic intervention to prevent or slow the disease process.

What other forms of genetic PD are there?

Other mutations causing highly penetrant ("Mendelian") hereditary parkinsonism are, like alpha-synuclein (PARK1) and parkin (PARK2) before them, shedding light on non-familial PD.

PARK4 was the designation given to the genetic locus associated with the Iowa kindred until it was discovered to be identical to PARK1[13].

PARK5 is ubiquitin carboxy terminal ligase 1 (UCHL-1) an enzyme involved in the ubiquitin-proteasome system for protein disposal. A point mutation causing a single amino acid substitution, ile93met, was found in two siblings with PD[36]. However, the statistical power of the disease-mutation association in that family is low and not fully accepted. A different variant in UCHL-1, ser18tyr, has been found, in a meta-analysis of 11 studies comprising 1,970 cases and 2,224 controls, to reduce the risk of PD by 16% in heterozygotes and by 29% in homozygotes[37].

PARK6 is PTEN-induced kinase-1, or PINK-1[38]. A mutation there was initially found in a Spanish family with autosomal recessive, young-onset PD and subsequently in a few other such families and individuals world-wide. Many mutations have since been identified in PINK-1, which is located on chromosome 1p36. It is the second-most-common known genetic cause of early-onset recessive PD, after PARK2. The enzyme is located in mitochondria and involved in preventing apoptosis, at least partly by preventing release of cytochrome C, an apoptotic signal, from damaged mitochondria[39].

PARK7, or DJ-1, maps very close to PARK6 at chromosome 1p36 but is clearly separate from it. Like PARK6, PARK7 is associated with autosomal recessive, early-onset PD[40]. It accounts for less than 1% of familial PD. DJ-1 sequesters

Daxx, a "death protein," in the nucleus, where it is prevented from initiating the apoptotic process in the cytoplasm [41]. As for the other recessively acting causes of PD, dysfunction of DJ-1 would act via a loss of function rather than by a toxic gain-of-function as is the case for a dominantly-acting gene mutation like PARK1. Like, PARK6, it corroborates the notion that modulation of apoptosis may be a route to PD prevention.

PARK8 is a dominantly-acting gene at chromosome 12q12 that, like PARK6, is a kinase [42,43]. Leucine-rich repeat kinase 2, or LRRK2 is also termed dardarin, from the Basque word for "tremor." The most common mutation, gly2019ser, occurred in 6% of families with autosomal dominant PD in one study [44]. The enzyme has functions other than phosphorylation and the mechanism of its PD association are only starting to be worked out, but may be related to regulation of parkin. Interestingly, PARK8 mutations are associated with a variety of histopathologic pictures, most of which feature Lewy bodies, but some have tau-positive lesions suggesting progressive supranuclear palsy, and some neuronal loss without inclusions. This suggests that PARK8 renders a specific anatomical area, the nigrostriatal system, vulnerable, but that other influences determine the mode of cell death.

For the five remaining PD-associated genes, an approximate location, but not a specific gene or mutation, have been identified via linkage to a known marker. PARK3 causes PD in a few families of northern European origin. It has been localized to chromosome 2p11-p13, the same region that has been found to be associated with sporadic PD in three large series of dually affected sibling pairs [45-48]. Such studies offer great power for identifying the general location of disease-causing mutations (but not, as yet, for identifying the precise gene or mutation). In two of these studies, PARK3 was associated not with the presence of PD, but with age of onset [47,48] PARK9, an autosomal recessive, teenage-onset form of PD is located at chromosome 1p36. It occurs in only one known family, in Jordan [49]. PARK10 was found at chromosome 1p32 via analysis of 117 patients from 51 Icelandic families [50]. PARK11, similarly, was found via analysis of a large number of unrelated families with multiple affected members, in this case a series ascertained by the Parkinson Study Group [51]. It is located at chromosome 2q36-q37. PARK12 was localized to chromosome Xq21-q25 by analysis of the same data set [52]. Two other groups have found the same localizations for a PD-associated gene in a large series of small families with PD, most of which are sibling pairs.

What about genes causing sporadic (that is, not obviously familial) PD?

Some "Mendelian" (that is, clearly dominant, recessive or X-linked) disorders can appear in sporadic form when the molecular dysfunction is mild, when the clinical onset of the disease occurs late in life, when there are few known, at-risk relatives, or when an ordinarily recessive defect is present in heterozygous form. The last condition applies to PARK2 and perhaps to PARK6.

Dozens of other genetic variants have been associated with sporadic PD, not via a total genome search, but by comparing the frequencies of alleles of candidate genes between patients (most of whom have no relatives with PD) and controls. This technique is prone to false positives and each newly announced association must be viewed in this light. Of the many suspect genetic variants identified in this way, four presently enjoy the strongest support.

One, located in the promoter region of alpha-synuclein, probably increases production of that protein, as occurs in families with multiplications of the alpha-synuclein region described above[53]. Another is in the gene encoding tau,[54] the microtubule-associated protein involved in Alzheimer's disease, progressive supranuclear palsy and other disorders. The mechanism here is not known, but may also have to do with excessive production of the protein. As mentioned above, aggregates of alpha-synuclein and tau stimulate aggregation of the other[27].

Finally, various detoxification genes have been variably associated with PD. These include the many components of the glutathione S-transferase (GST) and cytochrome P-450 systems and monoamine oxidase A and B. Each of these many enzymes detoxifies specific groups of toxic chemicals. While the data for none of these genes is unequivocal, this may be the result of failure to analyze the relevant subset of patients who are exposed to a specific toxin. For example, a variant in GST-P1 is over-represented not in PD in general, but in patients with PD who report exposure to pesticides[55].

What is the role of excessive oxidation in PD?

A molecule is "oxidized" when it donates an electron, and "reduced" when it receives an electron. Oxidation reactions can lead to the formation of free radicals, which are highly reactive, unstable molecules with an unpaired electron. Oxidative metabolism of dopamine produces hydrogen peroxide, which is normally rapidly cleared by protective mechanisms including the glutathione pathway. If protective mechanisms are overwhelmed, hydrogen peroxide can be reduced to form the highly reactive hydroxyl free radical, which can react with membrane lipids in the brain, leading to lipid peroxidation and cell damage. The brain may be rendered particularly vulnerable to oxidative damage by its disproportionate oxygen consumption, abundant lipid for peroxidation, and limited ability to regenerate [56]. An oxidative environment promotes the aggregation of alpha-synuclein [57,58], providing another possible route to neuronal degeneration.

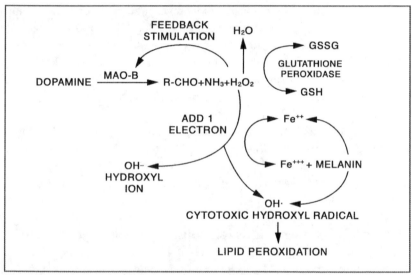

Figure 2.1. *Formation of cytotoxic hydroxyl radical. Dopamine's oxidative metabolism leads to the formation of hydrogen peroxide (H2O2). Hydrogen peroxide is normally cleared by glutathione. If protective mechanisms are overwhelmed, hydrogen peroxide can accept an electron to form hydroxyl ion (OH-) and cytotoxic hydroxyl radical (OH-). Melanin and iron may serve as electron donors and create site-specific oxidative stress.*

Are antioxidant protective enzymes abnormal in Parkinson's disease?

Parkinson's disease patients have decreased levels of reduced glutathione in the substantia nigra, without an increase in oxidized glutathione [39]. These findings are thought to be specific to Parkinson's disease, and are not observed in conditions such as multiple system atrophy. It is unclear whether decreased glutathione levels are caused by abnormalities in its synthesis or metabolism and the exact localization of the deficiency is also unknown. Decreased levels of reduced glutathione may compromise protective mechanisms, allowing hydrogen peroxide to become available to form hydroxyl radicals. GST, mentioned above in connection with toxin breakdown, also has anti-oxidant properties and is involved in glutathione metabolism. Its variability in PD may help explain the glutathione defect and the excess of oxidation products in PD brain.

What is the role of neuromelanin and iron in Parkinson's disease?

Oxidation reactions are facilitated by transition metals including iron, copper, and manganese. The brain contains a higher concentration of iron than any other metal, and it is probably essential for normal brain function. Iron accumulates in the normal brain until about age 20, after which time levels remain fairly constant. Iron is normally bound to the protein transferrin, which acts as a buffer to limit electron transfers. Parkinson's disease patients have increased iron levels in the substantia nigra pars compacta and decreased levels of transferrin, thus making iron more available for participation in oxidation reactions [60]. Neuromelanin in the substantia nigra has a high affinity for iron, and may serve as an electron source, thereby promoting the formation of free radicals [61]. The presence of neuromelanin may confer site-specific vulnerability on substantia nigra neurons. Iron also promotes the aggregation of alpha-synuclein, providing another explanation for the iron-PD association [23].

What is MPTP and what is its relationship to Parkinson's disease?

MPTP, or 1-methyl-4-phenyl-1,2,3,6-tetrahydropyridine, is a chemical that causes a clinical syndrome closely mimicking idiopathic Parkinson's disease. This was first observed in a chemist who was synthesizing illicit substances in his lab. He developed parkinsonism after intravenous injection of a mixture of 1-methyl-4-phenyl-4-hydroxypiperidine or MPPP, a potent meperidine analogue, and MPTP [62]. Autopsy revealed dopaminergic neuronal degeneration specifically within the substantia nigra.

Several other individuals who self-injected MPTP were later identified and examined [63]. Shortly after intravenous injection, these patients developed visual hallucinations, stiffness, limb jerking, and immobility. This stage was also marked by a sense of euphoria. Bradykinesia progressed for up to three weeks after injection. The ensuing chronic stage was marked by all of the motor features of Parkinson's disease, as well as some infrequent findings including eyelid apraxia, freezing, and dystonia.

Levodopa administration brought about marked improvement in parkinsonian signs and symptoms. Side effects of chronic dopamine replacement therapy such as dyskinesia occurred more rapidly than in idiopathic Parkinson's disease [63]. Autopsies revealed selective destruction of the dopaminergic neurons of the pars compacta of the substantia nigra. MPTP has since been utilized to create an excellent animal model of Parkinson's disease for research.

MPTP is actually a protoxin that is oxidized to the true toxin, MPP+, by the enzyme monoamine oxidase type B. MPP+ accumulates in mitochondria, and interferes with the function of Complex I of the respiratory chain. The extrinsic oxidation hypothesis suggests that an environmental protoxin is oxidized to a toxin that causes Parkinson's disease. Searches for such an environmental toxin have not identified a chemical that is likely to cause Parkinson's disease in idiopathic cases. Still, the identification of a chemical causing a syndrome so similar to Parkinson's disease is a landmark discovery that continues to provide new insights into possible etiologic mechanisms.

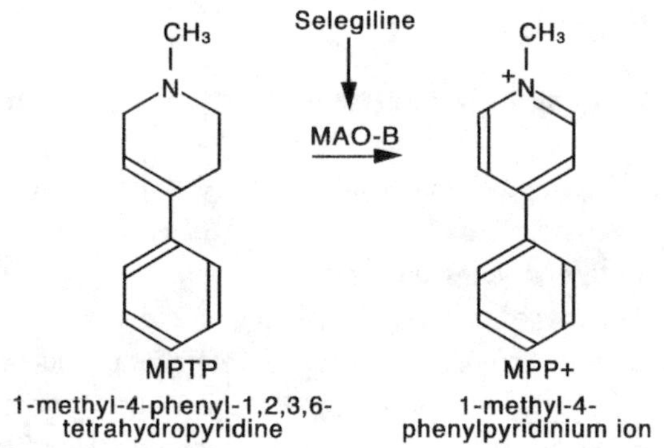

Figure 2.2. *Oxidation of MPTP to MPP+ is inhibited by selegiline, a selective inhibitor of MAO-B.*

What is the role of pesticides?

Soon after the identification of MPTP as a dopaminergic toxin, epidemiologists aware of the chemical resemblance of MPTP to some commonly used pesticides looked for occupational or residential risks associated with PD. They found a pesticide-PD association, but it is not clear that this is not merely a proxy for a different causal agent often encountered by the same rural population that tends to encounter pesticides [64]. Still, it is intriguing that rotenone and paraquat, two common pesticides, cause mitochondrial dysfunction and each promotes aggregation of alpha-synuclein [23]. Administration of rotenone to rodents produces alpha-synuclein aggregation and neuronal loss in a pattern similar to human PD [23].

What is the role of mitochondria in the pathogenesis of Parkinson's disease?

The toxic metabolite of MPTP, MPP+, inhibits complex I of the electron transport chain, causing a parkinsonian syndrome in affected individuals and laboratory animals [64]. This raises the question as to whether complex I is abnormal in idiopathic Parkinson's disease. Several laboratories have reported deficiencies of mitochondrial electron transport chain complex I in the substantia nigra of Parkinson's disease patients [65]. A blinded study examining platelet mitochondrial activity in early untreated Parkinson's disease patients and age- and sex-matched controls found lower complex I activity in platelet mitochondria in PD patients [66]. This suggests that chemical defects in Parkinson's disease may be widely expressed in the body and that the mitochondrial defect is genetically determined.

What is the role of smoking in the etiology of Parkinson's disease?

Cigarette smokers have approximately 40% less risk of developing PD relative to non-smokers [67]. The most plausible explanation is that smoking causes an induction of protective enzymes, but this is unproven. A competing hypothesis is that the very early stages of PD entail a deficiency in the dopaminergic addiction-reward system. Smoking or nicotine treatment provides no symptomatic benefit to patients with PD and of course, healthy nonsmokers, even those with a family history of PD, should not start smoking for the purpose of preventing PD.

What other environmental exposures may help cause Parkinson's disease?

Several aspects of rural living are associated with PD. Exposure to pesticides or herbicides, well water use, and farming experience have all been implicated in various surveys. Which of these, if any, is the actual culprit is unclear. A history of minor head trauma is also more common in PD [64]. Coffee drinking reduces PD risk by about 30%, possibly on the basis of adenosine receptor blockade [68].

Welding has been suggested to be associated with PD, but the data are still being evaluated. The association, if it exists, may be via inhalation of metal fumes that enhance alpha-synuclein aggregation [69].

Is Parkinson's disease simply an acceleration of aging?

No. There is loss of dopamine neurons in the substantia nigra pars compacta in normal aging, but it is greatest in the medial ventral and dorsal tiers. In Parkinson's disease, neuronal loss in greatest in the lateral ventral tier followed by the medial ventral and dorsal tiers [70].

Even more convincing, there is important neuronal loss in the caudate and putamen in aging, while those neurons, the sites of the dopamine receptors in the nigrostriatal pathway, remain intact in PD. This could explain the failure of the bradykinesia of aging to respond to dopamine replacement with levodopa [71]. Furthermore, Lewy bodies, the pathologic hallmark of degenerating neurons in PD, do not occur in large numbers in normal aging.

Is there a role for viruses in the etiology of Parkinson's disease?

Suspicion that viruses might play a role in the pathogenesis of Parkinson's disease was prompted by the occurrence of postencephalitic parkinsonism (PEP) following the outbreak of encephalitis lethargica (von Economo's encephalitis) from 1917-1926. However, in PEP, the protein that aggregates abnormally is tau, not alpha-synuclein, and even as the incidence of PEP declined dramatically after the 1920's, the incidence of PD remained stable. Virologic studies performed on brains of Parkinson's disease patients using electron microscopy and immunofluorescent studies have failed to detect viral particles or antibodies [72]. An old theory linking PD with the influenza pandemic of 1918 has also been thoroughly discredited.

How does all this fit together into a causative theory and provide clues for PD prevention?

We can combine these many points of evidence into a complex, tentative, general theory of the cause of "idiopathic" PD, shown in Figures 3 to 7. As can be seen from these figures, the current theory is that multiple cellular mechanisms participate. As more evidence accumulates, some of the components of the theory will receive greater emphasis, new ones will be added, and others may be discarded as irrelevant to the cause of more than a few cases. The relative importance of the components probably differs across individuals with PD. Linking the figures to one another is the common thread of alpha-synuclein aggregation.

The final, proximate cause of neuronal death may be apoptosis, or programmed cell death. If direct inhibition of apoptosis fails to prevent PD, then perhaps inhibition of alpha-synuclein aggregation will.

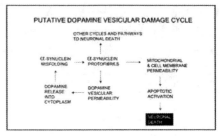

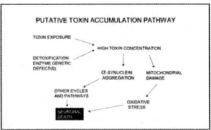

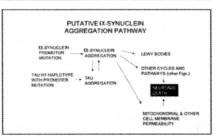

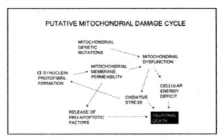

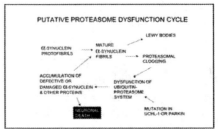

Figures 2.3 - 2.7.

CHAPTER 3

DIFFERENTIAL DIAGNOSIS OF PARKINSON'S DISEASE

Theresa A. Zesiewicz, Robert A. Hauser

The differential diagnosis of Parkinson's disease is vast. Causes of secondary Parkinsonism include medications and toxins, cerebrovascular disease, infection, trauma, metabolic abnormalities, and brain neoplasms (figure 3-1). The "atypical parkinsonisms" are a group of degenerative disorders with clinical features that include bradykinesia and rigidity, but differ from Parkinson's disease both pathologically and clinically. The atypical parkinsonisms are characterized clinically by lack of tremor, early speech and balance difficulty, and little or no response to dopamine medication therapy. This group of diseases includes progressive supranuclear palsy, corticobasal degeneration, and the multiple-system atrophies.

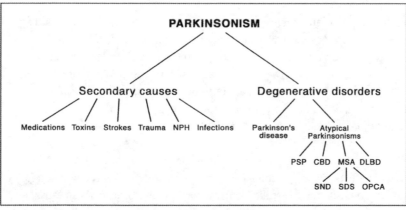

Figure 3.1. *The differential diagnosis of Parkinsonism.*

NPH=Normal Pressure Hydrocephalus　　*CBD=Corticobasal Degeneration*
SND=Striatonigral Degeneration　　*OPCA=Olivopontocerebellar Atrophy*
PSP=Progressive Supranuclear Palsy　　*MSA=Multiple System Atrophy*
SDS=Shy-Drager Syndrome　　*DLBD=Diffuse Lewy Body Disease*

The multiple system atrophies are marked clinically by a combination of extrapyramidal, pyramidal, autonomic, and cerebellar abnormalities. Included in the multiple system atrophies are striatonigral degeneration, olivopontocerebellar atrophy, and Shy-Drager syndrome.

This chapter will examine the differential diagnosis of Parkinson's disease, including characteristic features used to help recognize various diseases and possible therapies.

When should I be most suspicious that I am dealing with something other than Parkinson's disease?

One should always consider the differential diagnosis of Parkinson's disease before making a diagnosis. In all cases it is important to exclude the possibility of medication-induced parkinsonism. When dealing with young patients, one's index of suspicion for other disorders should be especially high as Parkinson's disease is generally a disease of older individuals. In patients with bradykinesia and rigidity, the combination of the absence of tremor and little or no response to dopaminergic medications greatly increases the likelihood that the correct diagnosis is not Parkinson's disease.

Which medications cause parkinsonism?

Many pharmacologic agents can produce features of parkinsonism, including tremor, bradykinesia, rigidity, shuffling gait, and speech disturbances. These include dopamine-blockers such as the neuroleptics and antiemetics, as well as dopamine depletors such as reserpine and tetrabenazine. The gastrointestinal motility drug metochlopramide has both peripheral and central dopamine antagonism, and is probably the most under recognized cause of medication-induced parkinsonism today.

Other drugs that can cause extrapyramidal signs include lithium[1], alpha-methyl-dopa[2], and some of the tricyclic antidepressants[3]. Antiepileptic medications can induce cerebellar symptoms[4] and valproic acid can cause tremor[5]. Patients presenting with parkinsonism who have recently taken any of these medications should be observed for at least six months off the medication before a diagnosis of Parkinson's disease is made[6].

Which toxins cause parkinsonism?

Toxins known to cause parkinsonian symptoms include manganese, carbon monoxide, methanol, ethanol, and MPTP or 1-methyl-4-phenyl-1, 2, 3, 6-tetrahydropyridine, a synthetic heroin derivative[7].

Which neurologic conditions mimic Parkinson's disease?

ARTERIOSCLEROTIC PARKINSONISM was first described by Critchley in the 1920's. "Vascular parkinsonism" is usually characterized clinically by bradykinesia and rigidity without tremor, and there may be other neurologic evidence of stroke[8]. Patients with multiple strokes may experience a step-wise progression of symptoms. An MRI should confirm the presence of cerebrovascular disease, although precise MRI criteria for a diagnosis of vascular parkinsonism are lacking. Tremor caused by cerebrovascular disease is uncommon, although there have been reports of unilateral tremor caused by vascular lesions in the thalamus[9]. Dystonia may also be caused by strokes involving the basal ganglia.

INFECTIONS, including viruses such as HIV, and tuberculosis can cause parkinsonian signs. Postencephalitic parkinsonism is an historic example of an infectious cause of parkinsonism. "Encephalitis lethargica" or "von Economo's disease" occurred in an epidemic from 1919-1926. It commonly affected young adults in their 20s and 30s, but also affected a substantial number of children[10]. Early symptoms included fever, mental changes, and neurologic deficits consistent with encephalitis. Mortality rates were high. Those who survived were left with various neurologic deficits in the chronic encephalitic phase.

Parkinsonism developed weeks to years after the acute phase[11]. Postencephalitic parkinsonism included bradykinesia and rigidity. Additional characteristic features were oculogyric crises with involuntary upward deviation of both eyes, and sleep rhythm disturbances. The parkinsonian features were often relatively stable and limited in progression. Pathologic changes were seen in the substantia nigra, subthalamic nucleus, and hypothalamus[10]. Very few postencephalitic parkinsonism patients are alive today owing to the more than eighty years that have elapsed since the outbreak of encephalitis lethargica.

TRAUMA can also cause parkinsonism. Boxers who endure repeated trauma to the head may develop a syndrome of dementia, parkinsonism, pyramidal, and cerebellar signs[12]. "Dementia pugilistica" refers to the cognitive changes boxers experience years after the trauma occurred. Multiple concussions cause diffuse axonal injury secondary to acceleration-deceleration forces affecting the brain. It is postulated that repeated head trauma may initiate dopamine neuron degeneration. Pathologically, there is a loss of pigmented neurons in the substantia nigra, in the absence of Lewy bodies. Neurofibrillary tangles without senile plaques are found in the cerebral cortex [13].

NORMAL PRESSURE HYDROCEPHALUS is an acquired condition leading to changes in mentation, gait disturbances, and urinary incontinence. Patients develop bradykinesia without tremor. Gait apraxia mimics the shuffling gait of Parkinson's disease. The diagnosis is made by a combination of clinical and imaging findings. MRI demonstrates hydrocephalus with the lateral ventricles dilated out of proportion to the cortical sulci and Sylvian fissures. Radionuclide cisternagram may demonstrate slow clearance of CSF. Some, but not all, patients will respond to shunting. Unfortunately, it is not currently possible to predict which patients will respond.

TUMORS and other mass lesions can occasionally cause parkinsonian features. This can be due to direct compression of the nigrostriatal tract by tumor or by stretching due to hydrocephalus.

What neurologic diseases are in the differential diagnosis of Parkinson's disease?

Essential Tremor (familial tremor) is characterized by a postural tremor of the upper extremities not caused by a pharmacologic agent [14]. The disease can begin as early as childhood and transmission is autosomal dominant with approximately 70% of patients reporting a family history of tremor. The tremor is predominantly postural, often with a kinetic component. The postural component is observed with the arms outstretched and the kinetic component with the arms in motion such as when performing the finger-to-nose test. Tremor frequency is often higher than that of Parkinson's disease, with a range of 4 to 12 Hz [15].

Essential tremor usually involves the upper extremities, is relatively symmetric, and is best seen with the arms outstretched, resulting in a flexion-extension or pronation-supination movement of the hands. The tremor slowly worsens over time [16]. Stressful activities transiently increase the amplitude of the tremor, and ingestion of alcohol may temporarily reduce it. The arms are usually affected, while the legs and trunk are normally spared. Essential tremor commonly includes a head or voice tremor, whereas tongue, jaw, and lip tremors are more characteristic of Parkinson's disease.

Other clinical manifestations of Parkinson's disease such as bradykinesia and rigidity are not present in essential tremor. Fifty to eighty percent of patients diagnosed with essential tremor will experience a good clinical response to medications such as propranolol or primidone [17]. However, this response is somewhat non-specific as the tremor of Parkinson's disease may also respond to these medications. However, essential tremor does not respond to dopamine medications.

Essential tremor is often mistaken for Parkinson's disease as it can be somewhat asymmetric and can sometimes be seen with the arms in a position of rest. For this reason we do not make a diagnosis of Parkinson's disease in a patient who only has tremor, although a classic parkinsonian rest tremor does suggest the possibility that other cardinal features will develop over time. A five-year history of bilateral upper extremity tremor without the emergence of bradykinesia or rigidity suggests a diagnosis of essential tremor rather than Parkinson's disease.

WILSON'S DISEASE is a disorder of copper metabolism transmitted by autosomal recessive inheritance [18]. The responsible gene has been mapped to the long arm of chromosome 13. Wilson's disease is a disease of children, adolescents, and young adults. Symptoms rarely occur before age six or after age 40. In children, hepatobiliary symptoms predominate whereas in adolescents and young adults neuropsychiatric symptoms are the rule. The exact etiology is unknown but the biology results in a positive copper balance. Free copper deposits in the liver and brain, leading to cirrhosis and neuropsychiatric features. The disease is associated with low levels of ceruloplasmin, a serum protein responsible for binding copper, increased liver copper concentration, and increased urinary copper excretion.

Patients may present with tremor (often of a "wing-beating" variety), dysarthria, rigidity, bradykinesia, dystonia and psychiatric disturbances. A pathognomonic feature of the neuropsychiatric form of the disease is the presence of Kayser-Fleischer rings, a brownish discoloration of the peripheral cornea seen on slit lamp examination of the eyes. Any young patient presenting with an unexplained tremor, parkinsonism, or abnormal movements should receive a screening evaluation for Wilson's disease. This includes a serum ceruloplasmin level determination, measurement of urinary copper, and an ophthalmologic examination. Treatment includes decreasing the amount of copper in the diet, as well as use of a copper chelator, such as D-penicillamine. Wilson's disease is one of the few potentially devastating genetic diseases for which there are effective medical therapies. A high index of suspicion is required to diagnose this treatable disorder.

HALLERVORDEN-SPATZ SYNDROME is a disease of the young, from infancy to young adulthood. Most cases are thought to be transmitted by autosomal recessive inheritance. Patients present with extrapyramidal symptoms including dystonia, rigidity, choreoathetosis and tremor, corticospinal tract signs, and dementia. The clinical course is progressive, leading to death. Abnormal accumulation of iron has been found in the GP and SNr of affected individuals. This massive accumulation of iron often produces prominent signal hypointensity in the GP and SNr on high field strength T2-weighted MRI. There is currently no effective treatment.

Neuroacanthocytosis is characterized clinically by adult onset, progressive orofacial dyskinesia, chorea and dystonia of the limbs, and a predominantly motor polyneuropathy with amyotrophy[19]. Additional signs can include seizures, parkinsonism, areflexia, and variable psychiatric disturbances with or without dementia. Some patients experience a progressive akinetic-rigid syndrome that gradually replaces the hyperkinetic features[20]. It is usually transmitted by autosomal recessive inheritance although autosomal dominant, x-linked, and sporadic cases have also been reported.

Characteristic laboratory findings include increased levels of serum creatinine kinase and acanthocytes, erythrocytes with irregular spines projecting from the cell surface, presumably caused by a defect in membrane lipids. Pathology findings include atrophy of the caudate nuclei and putamena, and occasionally of the globi pallidi. Anterior horn cell loss may be present as well as chronic axonal neuropathy with demyelination[21]. Treatment is limited to symptomatic therapy with neuroleptics for chorea and anticonvulsants for seizures. Patients with bradykinesia or rigidity may respond to dopaminergic therapy.

Huntington's Disease is a degenerative, autosomal-dominant disorder characterized by chorea, personality changes, and dementia[22]. Onset usually occurs in middle age, although some cases begin in childhood or adolescence[23]. Huntington's disease is caused by an increased number of trinucleotide (CAG) repeats in the gene on the short arm of chromosome 4[24]. The worldwide prevalence is 5-10 per 100,000. There is no therapy known to slow the progression of the disease and death commonly occurs 15-20 years after onset of symptoms.

Family members may notice that an affected patient has become short-tempered and depressed. He or she may be unable to sit still for any period of time, and may develop involuntary movements of the limbs, with decreased ocular saccades. Eventually, involuntary choreiform movements emerge, along with dementia. Atrophy of the caudate and putamen may be seen on imaging studies. Suicide is fairly common if depression is present, and patients are usually confined to a nursing home in the later stages. Therapy is limited to symptomatic treatment using antidepressants for depression and neuroleptics or other agents when necessary to control chorea [25]. Neuroleptics reduce chorea but often at the expense of side effects including apathy, sedation, akathisia, and parkinsonism. They should be reserved for those patients in whom chorea impairs function or self-care.

Five to ten percent of patients have juvenile Huntington's disease with onset before age twenty. Juvenile Huntington's disease is usually manifest by parkinsonian symptoms including bradykinesia, rigidity, and sometimes tremor. Dystonia and impaired eye movements may predominate and patients may have seizures. Ninety percent of juvenile Huntington's disease patients inherit the gene from an affected father, due to the large increase in the number of triplet repeats that can occur during spermatogenesis. Bradykinesia and rigidity may improve with levodopa therapy.

What are the "atypical parkinsonisms"?

The atypical parkinsonisms are a group of adult-onset progressive neurologic disorders that are characterized by bradykinesia and rigidity clinically and more widespread neuronal degeneration than Parkinson's disease histologically. The atypical parkinsonisms include progressive supranuclear palsy, corticobasal degeneration, and the multiple system atrophies. The multiple system atrophies are a group of closely related disorders that include degeneration in the extrapyramidal, pyramidal, autonomic, and cerebellar systems.

How can I clinically recognize the atypical parkinsonisms?

In contrast to Parkinson's disease, the atypical parkinsonisms are generally symmetric, lack resting tremor, and respond little, if at all, to dopaminergic medications. There is usually early speech and balance impairment, and rigidity may be greater in the neck than the extremities. Some of the atypical parkinsonisms are associated with characteristic clinical signs that aid in their identification. The most important diagnostic distinction is between Parkinson's disease, which responds well to medical therapy, and the atypical parkinsonisms that do not.

What is progressive supranuclear palsy?

PROGRESSIVE SUPRANUCLEAR PALSY (PSP) is one of the atypical parkinsonisms or "parkinson plus" syndromes. It was originally described by Steele, Richardson, and Olszewski[26], and has a prevalence of approximately 7/100,000 individuals over age 55[27]. PSP has a later mean age of onset than Parkinson's disease, and most patients are in their sixties or seventies. PSP is marked by bradykinesia and rigidity, postural instability, dysarthria, gait disturbances, and speech and swallowing difficulty[28]. Tremor is unusual. The characteristic clinical sign of PSP is a supranuclear gaze palsy. This refers to the fact that the patient is unable to voluntarily move the eyes, but the eyes move normally in response to passive head movements (oculocephalic testing). This finding implies that the difficulty must be above the nuclei that produce eye movements, and hence it is called supranuclear palsy. Downgaze is first affected followed by upgaze and later horizontal gaze. Slow saccade velocity may precede limitations of eye movements[28].

Some patients may complain of difficulty looking down, or note blurred vision but many have no visual complaints. Blink rate is markedly reduced and there may be "ocular stare" with the upper eyelids resting above the irises. Some patients exhibit neck extension rather than the stooped posture of Parkinson's disease. When turning, patients may cross their feet rather than turning "en bloc" as do Parkinson's disease patients. Falling due to imbalance occurs relatively early, often within a year or two of symptom onset. Blepharospasm and other focal dystonias are not unusual[29]. Dementia similar to that seen in patients with frontal lobe dysfunction is relatively common, particularly later in the disease[30]. On pathology examination, neuronal degeneration is present in the pallidum, subthalamic nucleus, and other areas. Lewy bodies are absent.

What are the multiple-system atrophies?

MULTIPLE SYSTEM ATROPHIES (MSA) refer to neurodegenerative diseases that are characterized by some or all of the following features: parkinsonism, autonomic and cerebellar dysfunction, and pyramidal signs[31a,32]. The multiple-system atrophies (MSAs) include striatonigral degeneration, Shy-Drager syndrome, and olivopontocerebellar atrophy[31b,32]. Neuronal degeneration is much more widespread than in Parkinson's disease, and may include the striatum, substantia nigra, olives, pons, cerebellum, and spinal cord [32]. Lewy bodies are absent but inclusions composed of alpha synuclein can be found in glial cells.

The early onset of frequent falling, coupled with cerebellar, pyramidal, or autonomic dysfunction usually suggests a diagnosis of MSA. Resting tremor is unusual but may be seen in some cases. Speech is more severely affected in MSA than in Parkinson's disease, and patients often develop early and dramatic hypophonia. Abnormal eye movements consisting of slow saccades or impaired convergence may be present. Myoclonic jerks may also occur. Response to dopaminergic therapy is poor and treatment consists of symptomatic and supportive care.

What is Shy-Drager syndrome?

SHY-DRAGER SYNDROME is an atypical parkinsonism characterized by prominent autonomic dysfunction. Clinical features of autonomic dysfunction may include orthostatic hypotension (or syncope), impotence, urinary incontinence and sweating abnormalities. Vocal cord paralysis, speech disturbances, sleep apnea, and psychiatric changes may also occur.

G. Milton Shy and Glenn Drager originally described a group of patients with orthostatic hypotension, urinary incontinence, loss of sweating, ocular palsies, iris atrophy, rigidity, impotence, and wasting of distal musculature with EMG findings suggestive of anterior horn cell involvement [33]. The disorder most commonly affects patients in their 50s to 70s, and is more common in men. Impotence is a common early manifestation in men, while lightheadedness is often the first noticed feature in women. The disease is progressive, and ultimately leads to death.

On pathology, marked gliosis is seen in the intermediolateral column of the spinal cord with changes noted in sympathetic ganglia. Cell degeneration is also seen in the inferior olivary nucleus, dorsal vagus nucleus, and substantia nigra pars compacta. Abnormalities may be seen in the cerebellum, Edinger-Westphal nucleus, oculomotor nucleus, and caudate nucleus. Noradrenergic neurons of brain and sympathetic ganglia are affected, with marked loss of tyrosine hydroxylase activity in the locus ceruleus. Dopamine-b-hydroxylase activity has also been found to be diminished in sympathetic ganglia [34].

Dopaminergic medications are usually not of benefit and may worsen symptoms of orthostasis [35]. Symptomatic therapy for orthostatic hypotension may be helpful.

What is olivopontocerebellar atrophy?

OLIVOPONTOCEREBELLAR ATROPHY (OPCA) is characterized by parkinsonism and cerebellar dysfunction [36]. The disease may occur by autosomal dominant inheritance or sporadically, and may affect individuals from infancy through the sixth decade. Patients may present with gait ataxia, extrapyramidal and pyramidal signs, and sphincter disturbances. Familial cases usually begin at a younger age, progress more slowly, and exhibit less autonomic failure than sporadic cases.

Cerebellar abnormalities are usually the presenting feature of dominantly inherited forms of OPCA. Parkinsonian symptoms may be early or late manifestations [37]. Speech difficulties, swallowing impairment, dementia, and visual disturbances may also occur. Response to dopaminergic therapy is usually poor. Neuronal degeneration occurs in the pons, inferior olives, and cerebellar cortex as well as the substantia nigra, pyramidal tracts, and thalamus [38]. CT and MRI typically show cerebellar atrophy, with widened cerebellopontine cisterns [39].

What is striatonigral degeneration?

Striatonigral degeneration [40] is an adult-onset progressive, symmetric, bradykinetic-rigid disorder characterized by early falling, speech and swallowing difficulties. Hyperreflexia and sleep apnea may be present. Resting tremor is much less common than in Parkinson's disease, and response to dopaminergic therapy is poor. Age at onset is comparable to that of Parkinson's disease, but progression of disability is much more rapid. On pathology, neuronal loss is found in the striatum, with widespread changes also noted elsewhere [41]. Cell loss is also seen in the substantia nigra, but Lewy bodies are rare.

What is corticobasal ganglionic degeneration?

Corticobasal ganglionic degeneration is a progressive, adult-onset bradykinetic-rigid syndrome characterized by the presence of both parkinsonism and cortical dysfunction. In contrast to other atypical parkinsonisms, there is often marked asymmetry. Parkinsonian features include bradykinesia and asymmetric limb rigidity. Cortical features include apraxia and cortical sensory loss [42,43]. Patients may have involuntary mirror movements or levitation of an arm ("alien-limb" phenomenon). Associated features include postural instability, hyperreflexia, focal reflex myoclonus, and apraxia of eye movement. On pathology the disease is characterized by asymmetric atrophy of the frontal and parietal lobes, and substantia nigra, with neuronal achromasia and large, swollen appearing neurons [44]. There is no treatment known to be effective for this disorder. Injections of botulinum toxin are sometimes useful to reduce marked rigidity in an arm or hand but do not improve limb function.

What is Lewy body disease?

Lewy body disease (LBD) is an atypical parkinsonism characterized by dementia, and autonomic abnormalities. It is marked pathologically by cortical and brainstem Lewy bodies [45,46]. Symptoms include dementia often with fluctuations in cognitive state, hallucinations, syncopal episodes, and depression. Dementia usually occurs early in the disease, and parkinsonian features follow. Dysphasia and agnosia may also occur. On pathology, Lewy bodies are found in the cortex, limbus, hypothalamus, and brainstem nuclei. Dopamine medications may improve parkinsonian features but may also induce or worsen hallucinations.

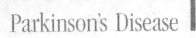

CHAPTER 4

MOTOR FEATURES OF PARKINSON'S DISEASE

Theresa A. Zesiewicz, Robert A. Hauser

What are the cardinal features of Parkinson's disease?

The four cardinal signs of Parkinson's disease are resting tremor, rigidity, bradykinesia, and postural instability. Tremor is the oscillation of a body part about a joint and is commonly observed as "shaking back and forth." Rigidity refers to increased resistance (stiffness) when a joint is passively flexed and extended. Bradykinesia means slowness of movement. It also encompasses decreased spontaneous movements and decreased amplitude of movement.

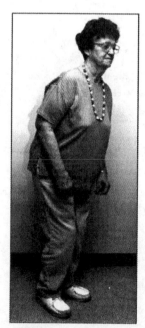

Figure 4.1. *Characteristic flexed posture of a patient with Parkinson's disease. (used with permission)*

Postural instability refers to imbalance and in contrast to the first three cardinal features does not emerge until late in the disease. The most common initial finding is an asymmetric resting tremor although about twenty percent of patients first experience clumsiness of a hand[1].

What other clinical features are associated with Parkinson's disease?

Patients with early Parkinson's disease often notice difficulty with fine coordinated movements and daily tasks become more difficult. There may be more difficulty buttoning shirts, combing one's hair, or playing golf. The first-affected arm may not swing fully when walking, and the foot on the same side may scuff or drag along the floor. Handwriting may become small (micrographia) and cramped. Family members may notice decreased facial expression (masked face). Speech may become soft (hypophonia) and monotonal.

Axial posture becomes progressively flexed and strides are shortened (figure 4.1), thereby causing a "shuffling" gait. The patient may eventually notice drooling and have difficulty swallowing foods. Pain may occur in an affected limb, sometimes leading to an erroneous diagnosis of arthritis or bursitis. Often this aching pain involves a large muscle group on one side of the body, commonly the calf. This can be accompanied by movement (dystonia) in the leg with the foot or toes turning down or in. Patients may notice a change in the taste of food caused by a lack of smell (anosmia). Depression can occur at any time throughout the disease. Symptoms of autonomic dysfunction include constipation, urinary frequency, sweating abnormalities, dermatitis, and sexual dysfunction. Patients may also experience sleep disturbances. Dementia may emerge over many years.

How does one make the diagnosis of Parkinson's disease?

The best clinical predictors of a pathology diagnosis of Parkinson's disease are:

a. asymmetry of onset

b. presence of resting tremor

c. good response to dopamine medication therapy.

The clinical diagnosis of Parkinson's disease is made by evaluation of the patient's history, neurologic examination, and response to dopamine replacement therapy. There are no blood tests that make the diagnosis and brain CT and MRI are typically unrevealing.

The following categories have been proposed for a clinical diagnosis of idiopathic Parkinson's disease [2]:

1. It is **POSSIBLE** that the patient has Parkinson's disease if one of the following is present: tremor (either resting or postural), rigidity, or bradykinesia.

2. It is **PROBABLE** that the patient has Parkinson's disease if two of the major features (resting tremor, rigidity, bradykinesia, or postural instability) are present, or if resting tremor, rigidity, or bradykinesia are asymmetric.

3. It is **DEFINITE** that the patient has Parkinson's disease if three of the major features are present, or if two of the features are present with one of them presenting asymmetrically.

Causes of secondary parkinsonism are excluded before a diagnosis of idiopathic Parkinson's disease is made (see chapter 3). These include medications, cerebrovascular disease, toxins, infections, and metabolic abnormalities. Other degenerative disorders (Creutzfeld-Jacob disease, Gerstmann-Straussler syndrome, Wilson's disease, Huntington's disease, neuroacanthocytosis), postencephalitic, posttraumatic and other conditions (normal pressure hydrocephalus) must also be excluded.

How reliable is a diagnosis of Parkinson's disease?

Two clinical-pathological studies found that 25% of patients diagnosed by neurologists with PD during life actually had other diagnoses based on autopsy findings. Autopsy evaluations in these patients were consistent with striatonigral degeneration, progressive supranuclear palsy, multi-infarct dementia, and Alzheimer's disease [3-5]. Interestingly, two-thirds of misdiagnosed patients reported a good to excellent response to levodopa, although the true extent of their response is not known.

It is very important to determine if parkinsonian symptoms including tremor, rigidity and bradykinesia truly improve with levodopa therapy. A meaningful (>50%) and sustained improvement in parkinsonian signs is thought to be a strong indicator of a pathology diagnosis of PD, but non-specific, unsustained or slight improvement is not. Fortunately, misdiagnosis based on clinical presentation and response to medication rarely causes a missed opportunity for improvement, as most mimickers of PD do not respond to any treatment. The exception to this is Wilson's disease (see chapter 3), which does require treatment to avoid irreversible damage.

What are the clinical characteristics of the tremor of Parkinson's disease?

Resting tremor is the most common presenting feature of Parkinson's disease, affecting almost seventy percent of patients [1]. It may be present in one or more limbs and is usually asymmetric. Tremor is typically present when the limb is at rest, but may also be seen with the limb in a position of postural maintenance (e.g., with the arms outstretched).

The characteristic tremor is a "pill-rolling" movement of the fingers or flexion/extension of the fingers or wrist. The frequency of the tremor is usually four to five cycles per second. The amplitude is quite variable and may change from minute to minute. The amplitude commonly increases in periods of stress such as

UK Parkinson's Disease Society Brain Bank clinical diagnostic criteria

Inclusion criteria	Exclusion criteria	Supportive criteria
Bradykinesia (slowness of initiation of voluntary movement with progressive reduction in speed and amplitude of repetitive actions)	History of repeated strokes with stepwise progression of parkinsonian features	(Three or more required for diagnosis of definite PD)
	History of repeated head injury	Unilateral onset
	History of definite encephalitis	Resting tremor present
And at least one of the following:	Oculogyric crises	Progressive disorder
Muscular rigidity	Neuroleptic treatment at onset of symptoms	Persistent asymmetry affecting side of onset most
4-6 Hz rest tremor	More than one affected relative	Excellent response (70-100%) to levodopa
Postural instability not caused by primary visual, vestibular, cerebellar, or proprioceptive dysfunction	Sustained remission	Severe levodopa-induced chorea
	Strictly unilateral features after 3 yr	Levodopa response for 5 yr or more
	Supranuclear gaze palsy	Clinical course of 10 yr or more
	Cerebellar signs	
	Early severe autonomic involvement	
	Early severe dementia with disturbances of memory, language, and praxis	
	Babinski sign	
	Presence of cerebral tumour or communicating hydrocephalus on CT scan	
	Negative response to large doses of levodopa (if malabsorption excluded)	
	MPTP exposure	

Table 4.1. *Hughes, AJ, Daniel SE, Kilford L Lees, AJ, Diagnostic criteria for Parkinson's disease, Journal of Neurology, Neurosurgery and Psychiatry, 1992, 55, 181-184, reproduced with permission from the BMJ Publishing Group.*

when the patient is asked to perform a cognitive task. Like most tremors, it disappears during sleep. The resting tremor of Parkinson's disease can be difficult to treat because of its variable response to medication therapy.

What is akinesia?

Akinesia literally means "lack of movement". In clinical use, it is synonymous with bradykinesia. These terms refer to slowness in the initiation and execution of movement. Parkinson's disease patients have longer reaction times coupled with an element of inattention that adds to their "slowness". This difficulty with movement is often described as the most disabling feature of the disease.

How does akinesia differ from akathisia?

Akathisia refers to a compulsion to move about and is commonly expressed as an inability to remain seated[8]. The initial stages of akathisia involve an inner feeling of restlessness, followed by the need to move. Unlike levodopa-induced dyskinesia, which is comprised of involuntary choreiform (random twisting, turning) movements, akathisia does not involve abnormal types of movement but rather an increased quantity of normal movements. Patients may march in place, pace back and forth, or perform repetitive movements of the limbs. Its exact etiology is unknown but is probably related to insufficient dopamine innervation. It is somewhat uncommon in Parkinson's disease, but is much more common in psychiatric patients.

In psychiatric patients, akathisia is commonly induced by anti-psychotic medications. In this setting, akathisia may be difficult to differentiate from the restlessness of psychotic agitation. Treatment of akathisia involves reduction of anti-dopaminergic medication, or the possible use of anticholinergics, antihistamines, or dopaminergic medications. Some studies have found beta-blockers to be helpful[3].

How do young and old onset Parkinson's disease patients differ?

Five to ten percent of Parkinson's disease patients experience onset of symptoms before age forty[9]. Patients who develop PD under age 21 are considered "juvenile PD" patients, while those who develop the disease from age 21 through 40 are said to have "young onset PD (YOPD)". The prevalence of PD in patients under 40 is generally estimated at 0-0.8 per 100,000 [3-5,10,11], although some studies found a prevalence rate as high as 4.7/100,000 [12,13].

Schrag et al. examined 139 YOPD patients, and found that all developed motor fluctuations and dyskinesia by 10 years post-diagnosis. Mortality risk was double that of the normal population. The median survival was 27 years for PD patients with disease onset from 36-39 years, and 35 years for patients with disease onset from 22-35 years. Cognitive impairment occurred in only 19% of patients[11].

A young patient who presents with parkinsonian features warrants a careful screen to rule out secondary causes of parkinsonism, especially those that are potentially treatable, such as Wilson's disease. Young onset Parkinson's disease patients are usually quite responsive to dopamine replacement therapy, have less dementia, and more readily develop levodopa-induced dyskinesias than their older counterparts[14]. Older patients are more likely to develop progressive bradykinesia that responds only partially to levodopa, and more likely to develop dementia.

How common are neuropsychiatric disturbances in Parkinson's disease?

In one sample of 139 PD patients in Norway, at least one "psychiatric" symptom was reported in 61% of patients. The most common psychiatric manifestations are depression (38%) and hallucinations (27%). Less common symptoms are euphoria and disinhibition[15]. Other studies have reported prevalence rates of psychosis in PD ranging from 6% to 40%, including visual hallucinations, delusions, dysphoria, mania, delirium, and abnormal sexual behavior[116-18].

What are the stages of Parkinson's disease?

One way to describe the severity of Parkinson's disease is the Hoehn and Yahr scale, developed by Margaret Hoehn and Melvin Yahr in the 1960s[9]. This scale describes five "stages" of Parkinson's disease. Progression on the scale reflects worsening disease severity but is not a linear indicator of disease progression[19].

Stage I:
Unilateral features of Parkinson's disease, including the major features of tremor, rigidity, or bradykinesia.

Stage II:
Bilateral features mentioned above, along with possible speech abnormalities, decreased posture, and abnormal gait.

Stage III:
Worsening bilateral features of Parkinson's disease, along with balance difficulties. Patients are still able to function independently.

Stage IV:
Patients are unable to live alone or independently.

Stage V:
Patients need wheelchair assistance, or are unable to get out of bed.

Disease corresponding to stages IV and V was found in 37% and 42% of patients with disease duration of 10 and 15 years, respectively[19]. However, Hoehn and Yahr also found considerable variability; 34% of patients with a disease duration of 10 years or longer were still in stages I or II, reflecting the heterogeneity of the disease[19, 20].

The Movement Disorders Task Force evaluated the Hoehn & Yahr scale, and found that its strengths included its wide utilization and acceptance, while its weaknesses included the scale's non-linearity and mixing of impairment and disability[21]. It is now recommended that the scale be used for descriptions of demographic presentation of patient groups, and for eligibility criteria in research settings.

How are the signs and symptoms of Parkinson's disease assessed in research studies?

The most commonly employed research scale is the "Unified Parkinson Disease Rating Scale (UPDRS)". The UPDRS is commonly used in clinical trials to evaluate change in PD signs and symptoms over time. It includes:

1) Mentation, Behavior, and Mood,

2) Activities of Daily Living (ADL) and

3) Motor sections. Individual items are rated from 0 to 4. The first two sections are evaluated by interview and the motor section is rated by examination. The individual item scores are summed to arrive at subset scores for each section, and to generate a total score[22]. A total of 199 points are possible, with 0=best possible score and 199=worst possible score.

Unified Parkinson Disease Rating Scale (UPDRS)

I. Mentation, Behavior, Mood

Intellectual Impairment

0 None

1 Mild; consistent forgetfulness with partial recollection of events with no other difficulties

2 Moderate memory loss with disorientation and moderate difficulty handling complex problems; mild but definite impairment of function

3 Severe memory loss with disorientation to time and often to place, severe impairment with handling problems

4 Severe memory loss with orientation preserved to person only; unable to make judgements or solve problems; requires much help with personal care; cannot be left alone at all

Thought Disorder

0 None
1 Vivid dreams
2 "Benign" hallucination with insight retained
3 Occasional to frequent hallucinations or delusions; without insight, could interfere with daily activities
4 Persistent hallucination, delusions, or florid psychosis; not able to care for self

Depression

0 Not present
1 Periods of sadness or guilt greater than normal but never sustained for days or weeks
2 Sustained depression (one week or more)
3 Sustained depression with vegetative symptoms (insomnia, anorexia, weight loss, loss of interest)
4 Sustained depression with vegetative symptoms and suicidal thoughts

Motivation/Initiative

0 Normal
1 Less assertive than usual; more passive
2 Loss of initiative or disinterest in elective (nonroutine) activities
3 Loss of initiative or disinterest in day-to-day (routine) activities
4 Withdrawn; complete loss of motivation

II. Activities of Daily Living

Speech

0 Normal
1 Mildly affected; no difficulty being understood
2 Moderately affected; sometimes asked to repeat statements
3 Severely affected; frequently asked to repeat statements
4 Unintelligible most of time

Salivation

0 Normal
1 Slight but definite excess of saliva in mouth; may have nighttime drooling
2 Moderately excessive saliva; may have minimal drooling
3 Marked excess of saliva; some drooling
4 Marked drooling; requires constant use of tissue or handerkerchief

Swallowing

0 Normal
1 Rare choking
2 Occasional choking
3 Requires soft food
4 Requires nasogastric tube or gastrotomy feeding

Parkinson's Disease

Handwriting

- **0** Normal
- **1** Slightly small or slow
- **2** Moderately slow or small; all words are legible
- **3** Severely affected; not all words legible
- **4** The majority of the words are not legible

Cutting Food/Handing Utensils

- **0** Normal
- **1** Somewhat slow and clumsy, but no help needed
- **2** Can cut most foods, although clumsy and slow; some help needed
- **3** Food must be cut by someone, but can still feed slowly
- **4** Needs to be fed

Dressing

- **0** Normal
- **1** Somewhat slow, no help needed
- **2** Occasional assistance needed with buttoning, getting arms into sleeves
- **3** Considerable help required, but can do some things alone
- **4** Helpless

Hygiene

- **0** Normal
- **1** Somewhat slow, but no help needed
- **2** Needs help with shower or bathe, very slow in hygienic care
- **3** Requires assistance for washing, brushing teeth, combing hair, going to bathroom
- **4** Needs Foley catheter or other mechanical aids

Turning in bed and adjusting bedclothes

- **0** Normal
- **1** Somewhat slow and clumsy, but no help needed
- **2** Can turn alone or adjust sheets, but with great difficulty
- **3** Can initiate attempt, but cannot turn or adjust sheets alone
- **4** Helpless

Falling (unrelated to freezing)

0 None
1 Rare falls
2 Occasionally falls, less than once daily
3 Falls an average of once daily
4 Falls more than once daily

Freezing When Walking

0 None
1 Rare freezing when walking; may have start hesitation
2 Occasional freezing when walking
3 Frequent freezing; occasionally falls because of freezing s
4 Frequently falls because of freezing

Walking

0 Normal
1 Mild difficulty; may not swing arms or may tend to drag leg
2 Moderate difficulty, but requires little or no assistance
3 Severe disturbance of walking; requires assistance
4 Cannot walk at all, even with assist

Tremor

0 Absent
1 Slight and infrequently present
2 Moderate; bothersome to patient
3 Severe; interferes with many activities
4 Marked; interferes with most activities

Sensory Complaints Related to Parkinsonism

0 None
1 Occasionally has numbness, tingling, and mild aching
2 Frequently has numbness, tingling, or aching; not distressing
3 Frequent painful sensations
4 Excruciating pain

III. Motor Exam

Speech

- **0** Normal
- **1** Slight loss of expression, diction, and/or volume
- **2** Monotone, slurred but understandable, moderately impaired
- **3** Marked impairment, difficult to understand
- **4** Unintelligible

Facial Expression

- **0** Normal
- **1** Minimal hypomimia; could be normal "poker face"
- **2** Slight but definitely abnormal diminution of facial expression
- **3** Moderate hypomimia; lips are parted some of the time
- **4** Masked of fixed facies, with severe or complete loss of facial expression; lips parted ¼ inch (0.5 cm) or more

Tremor at Rest

- **0** Absent
- **1** Slight and infrequently present
- **2** Mild in amplitude and persistent, or moderate in amplitude but only intermittently present
- **3** Moderate in amplitude and present most of the time
- **4** Marked in amplitude and present most of the time

Action or Postural Tremor

- **0** Absent
- **1** Slight; present with action
- **2** Moderate in amplitude; present with action
- **3** Moderate in amplitude; present with posture-holding as well as with action
- **4** Marked in amplitude; interferes with feeding

Rigidity (judged on passive movement of major joints with patient relaxed in sitting position; "cogwheeling" to be ignore):

0 Absent
1 Slight or detectable only when activated by mirror or other movements
2 Mild to moderate
3 Marked but full range of motion easily achieved
4 Severe; range of motion achieved with difficulty

Finger taps (patient taps thumb with index finger in rapid succession with widest amplitude possible, each hand separately):

0 Normal
1 Mild slowing and/or reduction in amplitude
2 Moderately impaired; definite and early fatiguing; may have occasional arrests in movement
3 Severely impaired; frequent hesitation in initiating movements or arrest in ongoing movement
4 Can barely perform the task

Hand Movements (patient opens and closes hands in rapid succession with widest amplitude possible, each hand separately):

0 Normal
1 Mild slowing and/or reduction in amplitude
2 Moderately impaired; definite and early fatiguing; may have occasional arrests in movements
3 Severely impaired; frequent hesitation in initiating movements or arrests in ongoing movement
4 Can barely perform the task

Rapid Alternating Movements of hand (pronation-supination movements of hands, vertically or horizontally, with as large an amplitude as possible both hands simultaneously):

0 Normal
1 Mild slowing and/or reduction in amplitude
2 Moderately impaired; definite and early fatiguing; may have occasional arrests in movement
3 Severely impaired; frequent hesitation in initiating movements or arrests in ongoing movement
4 Can barely perform the task

Leg Agility (patient taps heel on ground in rapid succession, picking up entire leg; amplitude should be about three inches): tap heel on ground, amp should be three inches):

0 Normal
1 Mild slowing and/or reduction in amplitude
2 Moderately impaired; definite and early fatiguing; may have occasional arrests in movement
3 Severely impaired; frequent hesitation in initiating movements or arrests in ongoing movement.
4 Can barely perform the task

Arising From Chair (patient attempts to arise from a straight-backed wood or metal chair, with arms folded across cheast)

0 Normal
1 Slow, or may need more than one attempt
2 Pushes self up from arms of seat
3 Tends to fall back, may have to try more than one time but can get up without help
4 Unable to arise without help

Posture

- **0** Normal erect
- **1** Not quite erect, slightly stooped posture; could be normal for older person
- **2** Moderately stooped posture, definitely abnormal; can be slightly leaning to one side
- **3** Severely stooped posture with kyphosis; can be moderately leaning to one side
- **4** Marked flexion, with extreme abnormality of posture

Gait

- **0** Normal
- **1** Walks slowly; may shuffle with short steps, but not festination or propulsion
- **2** Walks with difficulty but requires little or no assistance; may have some festination, short steps, or propulsion
- **3** Severe disturbance of gait; requires assistance
- **4** Cannot walk at all, even with assistance

Postural Stability (response to sudden posterior displacement produced by pull on shoulders while patient is erect, with eyes open and feet slightly apart; patient is prepared):

- **0** Normal
- **1** Retropulsion, but recovers unaided
- **2** Absence of postural response; would fall if not caught by examiner
- **3** Very unstable; tends to lose balance spontaneously
- **4** Unable to stand without assistance

Body Bradykinesia and hypokinesia (combining slowness, hesitancy, decreased arm swing, small amplitude and poverty of movement in general):

- **0** None
- **1** Minimal slowness, could be normal, deliberate character
- **2** Mild slowness, giving movement a deliberate character; could be normal for some persons; possible reduced amplitude
- **3** Moderate slowness;poverty, or small amplitude of movement
- **4** Marked slowness; poverty, or small amplitude of movement

The Movement Disorders Task Force found that the UPDRS was widely utilized and comprehensively evaluated motor symptoms, but had inadequate instructions for raters, and failed to provide screening questions for many of the non-motor symptoms of PD[23]. The UPDRS is in the process of being revised, to include sections on non-motor experiences of daily living, motor experiences of daily living, objective motor examination, and assessment of motor complications.

How is disability rated in PD?

The Schwab and England Activities of Daily Living Scale is commonly used to assess disability in PD research[24].

Scoring can be performed by a rater or by the patient:

100% Completely independent; able to do all chores without slowness, difficulty, or impairment; essentially normal; unaware of any difficulty.

90% Completely independent; able to do all chores with some degree of slowness, difficulty and impairment; may take twice as long as normal; beginning to be aware of difficulty.

80% Completely independent in most chores; takes twice as long as normal; conscious of difficulty and slowness

70% Not completely independent; more difficulty with chores; takes three to four times as long as normal in some; must spend a large part of the day with chores

60% Some dependency; can do most chores, but exceedingly slowly and with considerable effort and errors; some chores impossible.

50% More dependent; needs help with half of chores, slower, etc.; difficulty with everything.

40% Very dependent; can assist with all chores but few alone.

30% With effort, now and then does a few chores alone or begins alone; much help needed.

20% Does nothing alone; can be a slight help with some chores; severe invalid

10% Totally dependent and helpless; complete invalid

0% Vegetative functions such as swallowing, bladder and bowel function are not functioning; bedridden

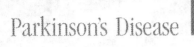

CHAPTER 5

COMPLICATIONS OF LONG-TERM THERAPY IN PD AND THE CONTINUOUS DOPAMINERGIC STIMULATION HYPOTHESIS

Theresa A. Zesiewicz, Robert A. Hauser

Levodopa, the precursor to dopamine, has been considered the "gold standard" of treatment for PD because it provides the greatest antiparkinsonian efficacy with the fewest short-term side effects. However, its use is complicated by the development of long-term side effects, specifically motor fluctuations and dyskinesias. The development of these long-term complications is thought to be due to a combination of disease progression and levodopa's short half-life.

Levodopa is usually administered with a peripheral dopadecarboxylase inhibitor (DDCI) such as carbidopa that reduces levodopa's metabolism in the blood and decreases nausea. The half-life of levodopa when administered with carbidopa is approximately 90 minutes. This means that levodopa is mostly cleared from the blood within four to six hours after administration.

What is the usual course of treated Parkinson's disease?

Patients usually experience good control of parkinsonian features when symptomatic therapy is first introduced. This "honeymoon" period is maintained for approximately three to five years into levodopa therapy[1,2]. Although levodopa has a short plasma half-life, patients initially experience a stable response through the day (figure 5.1). This is presumably due to the ability of remaining nigrostriatal neurons to generate dopamine from absorbed levodopa, store it intraneuronally and slowly release it into the synaptic cleft in a relatively normal fashion. Because there are 60-80% fewer dopamine neurons, the amount of dopamine released from each neuron is increased (increased dopamine turnover) in order to approximate the normal state.

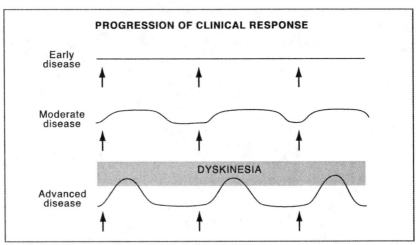

Figure 5.1. *Progression of clinical response in Parkinson's disease. Despite the short half-life of levodopa/DDCI, patients with early disease experience a sustained response through the day. As the disease progresses, patients begin to notice "wearing-off" fluctuations such that the benefit of levodopa/DDCI wears off after a few hours. Ultimately, clinical response fluctuates more and more closely in association with peripheral levadopa and patients develop choreiform dyskinesia when dopamine peaks. Arrows indicate times of levodopa/DDCI administration.*

Despite levodopa therapy, disability continues to progress over time[3]. This may be due to inadequate dopamine stimulation or degeneration of neurons downstream to dopamine receptors. Over the years there is a tendency to administer increasing amounts of dopaminergic medication in order to minimize functional disability.

Motor fluctuations begin to emerge as early as one to two years after initiation of levodopa therapy. Between approximately four and eight years, many patients experience motor fluctuations and dyskinesia that cause clinical disability. Patients begin to notice that whereas they used to be able to take standard levodopa/DDCI three or four times a day and still maintain a stable response, the benefit now lasts a few hours and then wears off. Patients may initially notice a short duration levodopa response of four to five hours. Over the next few years, the short duration response becomes more fleeting and benefit lasts only two to three hours. Over time, clinical status more and more closely fluctuates in concert with peripheral levodopa concentration[4]. Presumably, this is because as neuronal degeneration progresses, the capacity for surviving neurons to effectively store levodopa-derived dopamine diminishes.

During this time, many patients also develop peak-dose dyskinesias consisting of twisting, turning (choreiform) movements that occur when central (brain) dopamine levels are peaking [5,6]. This marks an important milestone in the treatment of Parkinson's disease because it limits the amount of dopaminergic therapy that can be provided. At this point, higher doses of dopaminergic therapy are likely to increase peak-dose dyskinesia. This "hypersensitivity" may result from exposing post-synaptic receptors to rapidly fluctuating levodopa-derived dopamine levels [4].

From five to 10 years into symptomatic therapy, much of the management of Parkinson's disease centers on titrating therapy to maximize ON time without dyskinesia. Too much dopaminergic therapy exacerbates peak-dose dyskinesias and too little dopaminergic therapy fails to bring about sufficient benefit. Despite optimal titration, many patients eight or more years into symptomatic therapy suffer with troublesome or disabling motor fluctuations and dyskinesia.

Some patients develop dementia as the disease progresses. As antiparkinsonian therapy can worsen confusion and hallucinations, the presence of cognitive dysfunction can also limit administration of medication to improve motor symptoms.

By 10 to 12 years or more, many patients have developed balance difficulty. This is another important milestone. True balance difficulty (postural imbalance) is not improved by any current antiparkinsonian therapy. Patients are then at risk for morbidity and mortality from falls. Immobility may place a patient at increased risk for infections and swallowing difficulty may increase the risk of aspiration and malnutrition. The cause of death in Parkinson's disease is often related to infection, injuries due to falls or other medical conditions such as stroke or heart attack.

Individual progression varies greatly. Some patients maintain relatively good function fifteen years into the disease and others experience meaningful disability within a few years.

What are the complications of long-term levodopa therapy in Parkinson's disease?

The complications of long-term therapy for Parkinson's disease include motor fluctuations and dyskinesia. Motor fluctuations consist of variations in clinical status that occurs over the course of a day. Dyskinesia refers to abnormal involuntary movements occurring in association with medication therapy.

What are the different types of motor fluctuations?

Wearing-off fluctuations are relatively predictable variations in motor function temporally associated with the timing of levodopa ingestion. When patients are initially placed on levodopa, they experience a stable clinical response through the day. However, after months to years, many patients experience benefit for only a few hours following levodopa ingestion. This is followed by a loss of benefit, or wearing- off. Symptom control can be regained by taking the next levodopa dose. In contrast, on-off fluctuations are rapid transitions (over seconds) between the ON and OFF states, seemingly unrelated to the timing of medication ingestion.

What are the ON and OFF states?

ON and OFF states can be identified in patients with motor fluctuations. ON refers to a patient's clinical status when medication is providing symptomatic benefit with regard to mobility, bradykinesia, and rigidity. OFF refers to a patient's status when symptomatic benefit has been lost over the preceding minutes or hours. Some patients also experience an intermediate state as re-emergence of tremor may precede loss of benefit for mobility, bradykinesia and rigidity.

Will my patient recognize motor fluctuations?

Patients with a stable response commonly report that they are unsure if they are experiencing motor fluctuations. In contrast, patients with motor fluctuations can usually identify these fluctuations without difficulty.

Does wearing-off affect other symptoms?

Although wearing-off was first defined as a wearing-off of benefit regarding motor symptoms, many patients also describe re-emergence of non-motor symptoms when levodopa wears off. These can include mood changes such as depression or anxiety, autonomic symptoms such as sweating, or cognitive changes such as cloudiness or slowing of thinking.

Is a worsening of tremor during periods of stress a type of motor fluctuation?

No. Patients commonly experience a transient increase in tremor (or dyskinesia) when emotionally activated. This phenomenon is not related to the pharmacokinetics of levodopa. Its cause is poorly understood.

What are the types of dyskinesia that occur in Parkinson's disease?

Involuntary abnormal movements associated with medication intake are categorized by the type of movement and the phase of the dosing cycle in which they occur. The three most common types of dyskinesia in Parkinson's disease are peak-dose dyskinesia, wearing-off dystonia, and diphasic dystonia/dyskinesia. They are often worse on the side of the body most affected and commonly emerge in patients who have had a good response to levodopa. The incidence is highest in young-onset patients [6].

Peak-dose dyskinesias are most common. They occur at the peak of the dosing cycle, when levodopa-derived dopamine is highest. They consist of choreiform, non-patterned, twisting, turning movements usually seen in the extremities, trunk, and head. They diminish when the levodopa dose is reduced and increase when the levodopa dose is raised.

Wearing-off dystonia occurs in association with low or falling dopamine levels [7]. It commonly occurs at night or in the morning prior to the first levodopa dose. It consists of involuntary, sustained muscle contractions and commonly occurs in the lower extremities causing foot inversion or plantar flexion. The dystonia may be associated with pain, particularly in the calf. It may respond to more sustained dopaminergic stimulation as provided by dopamine agonists, levodopa/carbidopa CR, or levodopa/carbidopa plus entacapone.

Diphasic dystonia/dyskinesia is relatively uncommon and occurs both when a patient is turning on and when wearing-off. It was originally called D-I-D dystonia/dyskinesia, indicating dystonia/dyskinesia was followed by improvement and then a return of dystonia/dyskinesia within a single dosing cycle [5]. It is often manifest as a combination of dystonia and chorea, and typically affects the lower extremities. Diphasic dyskinesia can be difficult to treat but usually an attempt is made to increase and smooth dopaminergic stimulation. D-I-D dyskinesia is often improved by deep brain stimulation of the globus pallidus or subthalamic nucleus (see chapter 10).

It can usually be assumed that chorea in the setting of treated Parkinson's disease represents peak-dose dyskinesia until proven otherwise because it is so common. The unqualified term dyskinesia in the context of Parkinson's disease usually refers to peak-dose dyskinesia.

How common are the long-term complications?

More than 50% of patients treated five years or longer may have motor fluctuations and dyskinesia [8]. Approximately 90% of patients develop motor fluctuations and dyskinesia by 15 years of disease.

Are these long-term complications caused by levodopa?

Normal individuals do not appear to develop motor fluctuations or dyskinesia if administered levodopa. The emergence of long-term complications occurs as a result of the combination of disease progression and levodopa administration.

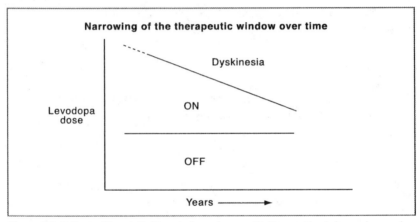

Figure 5.2. *Patients with early Parkinson's disease have a wide therapeutic window and respond well to a wide range of levodopa dosages. As the disease progresses, the therapeutic window narrows. Insufficient dosages in later disease may not bring about benefit (on). High dosages may cause choreiform dyskinesia.*

What is the "therapeutic window"?

Patients with both motor fluctuations and dyskinesia are said to have a therapeutic window. It lies above the threshold required to improve symptoms ("ON threshold") and below the threshold for peak-dose dyskinesia ("dyskinesia threshold"). When patients are ON without dyskinesia they are said to be in their therapeutic window.

What happens to the therapeutic window over time?

The therapeutic window appears to become smaller over time (figure 5.2). Much of the narrowing of the therapeutic window is due to a progressive lowering of the dyskinesia threshold. Once the window is sufficiently narrowed, it may be difficult to provide much ON time without dyskinesia and even optimal medication titration may do no more than provide a balance between OFF time and dyskinesia.

Which is worse, OFF time or dyskinesia?

Both OFF time and dyskinesia can be disabling. Most patients prefer dyskinesia to OFF time and most family members and physicians prefer for the patient to be OFF than have dyskinesia. It is important to listen to the patient and help them achieve the balance that they most prefer. Usually the goal is to maximize ON time while attempting to minimize troublesome or disabling dyskinesia. Having the patient fill out a diary divided into half-hour time periods can help the physician analyze the amount of OFF time and troublesome dyskinesia, and their relation to the timing of medication intake (figure 5.3) [9].

Are dopamine agonists associated with long-term complications?

Dopamine agonists are medications that act in the brain like dopamine. Unlike levodopa, they do not need to be metabolized and they are not stored in neurons. They act at dopamine receptors in the brain to provide benefit for PD symptoms. Currently available oral dopamine agonists have relatively long half-lives of at least six hours. They therefore provide relatively continuous dopamine stimulation. Their main limitation is that they are not as efficacious as levodopa to alleviate PD symptoms especially in moderate and advanced disease. Dopamine agonists are discussed in detail in the medication chapter.

PARKINSON'S DISEASE DIARY

NAME_____   DATE_____

Instructions: For each half-hour time period place one check mark to indicate your predominant status during most of that period.
ON = Time when medication is providing benefit with regard to mobility, slowness, and stiffness.
OFF = Time when medication has worn off and is no longer providing benefit with regard to mobility, slowness, and stiffness.
Dyskinesia = Involuntary twisting, turning movements. These movements are an effect of medication and occur during ON time.
Non-troublesome dyskinesia does not interfere with function or cause meaningful discomfort. Troublesome dyskinesia interferes with function or causes meaningful discomfort. Tremor is shaking back and forth and is not considered dyskinesia.

time	asleep	OFF	ON without dyskinesia	ON with non-troublesome dyskinesia	ON with troublesome dyskinesia	time	asleep	OFF	ON without dyskinesia	ON with non-troublesome dyskinesia	ON with troublesome dyskinesia
6:00 AM						6:00 PM					
:30						:30					
7:00 AM						7:00 PM					
:30						:30					
8:00 AM						8:00 PM					
:30						:30					
9:00 AM						9:00 PM					
:30						:30					
10:00 AM						10:00 PM					
:30						:30					
11:00 AM						11:00 PM					
:30						:30					
12:00 PM						12:00 AM					
:30						:30					
1:00 PM						1:00 AM					
:30						:30					
2:00 PM						2:00 AM					
:30						:30					
3:00 PM						3:00 AM					
:30						:30					
4:00 PM						4:00 AM					
:30						:30					
5:00 PM						5:00 AM					
:30						:30					

Figure 5.3. *Parkinson's disease diary.*

Motor fluctuations and dyskinesias are uncommon in patients on dopamine agonists alone (monotherapy). Agonists with long half-lives provide a relatively stable clinical response and it is unusual for a patient to experience motor fluctuations on these agents alone. However, patients with advanced disease do experience fluctuations when short-acting dopamine agonists such as apomorphine are administered. It is also uncommon for patients to experience dyskinesia on dopamine agonist monotherapy. In contrast, patients with peak-dose dyskinesia on levodopa commonly experience a worsening of dyskinesia when an agonist is added.

Thus, it is important to differentiate emergence of dyskinesia over time, from symptomatic worsening of dyskinesia in patients who already have (or are close to having) them. Dopamine agonists alone are associated with a low incidence of the emergence of dyskinesia. In patients with dyskinesia on levodopa, the addition of a dopamine agonist commonly causes symptomatic worsening of dyskinesia.

What is the Continuous Dopaminergic Stimulation (CDS) hypothesis?

Dopamine neurons in the brain normally release dopamine in a relatively stable, or continuous, manner. In early PD, remaining dopamine neurons take up levodopa, convert it to dopamine, store it, and slowly release it. However, over time as more dopamine neurons are lost, this storage and slow release capacity is lost. Fluctuations in plasma levodopa levels due to levodopa's short half-life can no longer be buffered and dopamine receptors in the brain are stimulated in an abnormal, pulsatile fashion.

The loss of intraneuronal storage and slow release capacity is expressed as a shortened duration of benefit from levodopa. Once this capacity is essentially lost, patients fluctuate in concert with levodopa fluctuations in plasma. It is thought that exposing dopamine receptors to abnormal, pulsatile stimulation causes changes that are expressed clinically as dyskinesia.

The Continuous Dopaminergic Stimulation (CDS) hypothesis states that treatment strategies that provide more continuous dopaminergic stimulation cause less motor fluctuations and dyskinesia.

What is the evidence in support of the CDS hypothesis?

Support for the CDS hypothesis comes from both animal and human studies. A large body of information comes from the MPTP monkey model of PD. Monkeys who receive MPTP, a dopamine neuron toxin, lose dopamine neurons and exhibit parkinsonian features (bradykinesia, rigidity). When treated with levodopa (which has a short half-life), they develop marked dyskinesia over several weeks. When levodopa is administered with entacapone, a COMT inhibitor that prolongs the levodopa half-life, the development of dyskinesia is reduced[10]. Further, MPTP monkeys treated with long-acting dopamine agonists develop little or no dyskinesia[11]. In contrast, short acting dopamine agonists induce dyskinesia but this can be prevented by continuous administration of the same agent.

In multiple clinical trials of PD patients, initial treatment with long acting dopamine agonists (pramipexole, ropinirole, cabergoline) has caused less motor fluctuations and dyskinesia than treatment with levodopa[12,13]. These studies are discussed in detail in the medication chapter.

Is the MPTP monkey model a good model of PD?

MPTP-treated monkeys are different from Parkinson's disease patients in a number of ways. They do not have Parkinson's disease and do not experience a progressive loss of dopamine neurons over many years. MPTP causes an acute loss of dopamine neurons and when relatively high doses of MPTP are given, the extent of dopamine neuron loss is similar to that seen in advanced PD. Because of this marked loss of dopamine neurons, MPTP monkeys treated with levodopa develop dyskinesia over a matter of weeks. The MPTP monkey model has thus far been highly predictive of the effects of dopamine treatments in PD patients. It is a very useful model to determine the extent to which dopaminergic treatments 1) improve parkinsonian signs, and 2) cause the development of dyskinesias.

How does this information impact medical management of PD?

Younger patients are more likely than older patients to develop motor fluctuations and dyskinesia, and have a longer time horizon over which they will be treated. In contrast, older patients are less likely to develop motor fluctuations and dyskinesia and may have a shorter time horizon for treatment. In addition, older individuals are more prone to short-term side effects such as hallucinations that are more common with dopamine agonists than levodopa.

One strategy that has emerged is to initiate dopaminergic therapy in younger patients (<65?) with a dopamine agonist and to add levodopa when the dopamine agonist alone is no longer sufficient. This strategy has been demonstrated to cause less motor fluctuations and dyskinesia. When levodopa needs to be added, entacapone can be introduced at the same time in an effort to continue to reduce the development of motor fluctuations and dyskinesia. This is supported by MPTP monkey studies, and is currently being evaluated in a clinical trial.

In older individuals (>70?), one might elect not to use dopamine agonists, but to introduce levodopa when treatment is required. As above, the use of entacapone to reduce the development of motor fluctuations and dyskinesia has been suggested by MPTP monkey studies and is being evaluated in PD patients.

For patients between approximately 65 and 70 years of age, a judgement can be made based on individual factors including general health and cognitive status.

What is freezing?

Freezing is a momentary inability to move one's feet during ambulation. Patients will describe that their feet feel stuck to the floor. Start-hesitation is freezing when a patient attempts to initiate ambulation. Freezing generally occurs late in Parkinson's disease and affects roughly one third of patients [14]. It occurs more frequently in those whose initial symptoms were gait-related. Turning or attempting to walk through a doorway may cause freezing and contribute to falls.

Freezing that occurs during OFF time is improved by medication changes that reduce OFF time. Freezing during ON time is poorly responsive to medication changes. Tricks or strategies such as attempting to march rather than walk, stepping over an object, or walking over masking tape placed across a walkway may be helpful. The development of freezing appears to be related to progression of disease but its underlying pathology is not known.

How do you conceptually classify Parkinson's disease patients?

We find it very helpful to classify patients based on their need for medication and whether they have developed motor complications. This classification system provides a shorthand description of where the patient is in the course of PD and helps dictate appropriate management. In addition, it often reflects eligibility used in clinical trials.

CLINICAL CLASSIFICATION OF PARKINSON'S DISEASE PATIENTS
© RA Hauser and TA Zesiewicz, 2000

Class 1:
Patient is not on any antiparkinsonian medications ("de novo").

Class 2:
Patient is on antiparkinsonian medication but not levodopa.

Class 3:
Patient is on levodopa and experiencing a stable response.

Class 4:
Patient is on levodopa and experiencing motor fluctuations without dyskinesia.

Class 5:
Patient is on levodopa and experiencing motor fluctuations and dyskinesia

Can non-motor symptoms of Parkinson's disease fluctuate like motor symptoms?

Non-motor symptoms of Parkinson's disease include fatigue, cognitive and mood disorders, sleeping problems, autonomic dysfunction, and abnormal sensations or pain. Non-motor symptoms of Parkinson's disease can fluctuate during the day with or without motor fluctuations, and can be disabling. In a prospective study based on a patient questionnaire, Witjas et al found that Parkinson's disease patients frequently experience non-motor symptoms, and that they are often associated with the motor OFF state.

Anxiety (66%), drenching sweats (64%), slowness of thinking (58%), and fatigue (56%) were the most frequently reported non-motor symptoms [15]. Anxiety and dyspnea correlated with greater levels of disability.

How can I determine whether I am experiencing wearing-off?

A 32-item Patient Questionnaire covering a wide range of motor and non-motor symptoms has been developed by a group of movement disorder experts to address the re-emergence of signs and symptoms that occur when the effect of levodopa wears off [16]. One study found that the presence of wearing-off symptoms was identified more frequently using this questionnaire than by standard assessments performed by movement disorder specialists. In clinical practice, the questionnaire can be used as a screening tool and starting point for discussion between patients and their doctor on possible need of treatment adjustment.

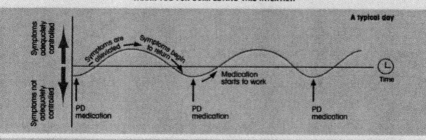

PATIENT SYMPTOMS QUESTIONNAIRE

You have been asked to complete this questionnaire to determine if you experience a relatively predictable worsening of your Parkinson's symptoms at different times during the day. This information is being gathered to help us gain a better understanding of how your symptoms change.

Some individuals experience a noticeable improvement in their Parkinson's symptoms after taking each dose of anti-parkinsonian medication. However, after a period of time some individuals experience a return of their symptoms before the next dose of medication has a chance to work.

These returning symptoms may include problems with movement and mobility (motor problems) or changes in feelings and sensations that can vary with the medication levels in your body (please refer to the figure).

Please complete this questionnaire to help us understand if you are experiencing any of the following symptoms that get better after taking your medication, but often reappear before your next dose.

THANK YOU FOR COMPLETING THIS INTERVIEW

Identification of motor and nonmotor wearing-off in Parkinson's disease: comparison of a patient questionaire versus a clinician assessment[16].

Stacy M, Bowron A, Guttman M, Hauser R, Hughes K, Larsen JP, LeWitt P, Oertel W, Quinn N, Sethi K, Stocchi F. Mov Disord 2005;20:726-733.

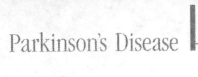

CHAPTER 6

MEDICATIONS FOR THE TREATMENT OF PARKINSON'S DISEASE

Theresa A. Zesiewicz, Robert A. Hauser

When did the modern era of Parkinson's disease treatment begin?

The discovery that Parkinson's disease is associated with a striatal dopamine deficiency created new possibilities for therapeutic approaches beginning in the late 1960s. Until then, anticholinergic medications were the principal treatment and results were disappointing. Patients were subsequently found to experience dramatic benefit when placed on the dopamine precursor, levodopa [1]. Today, levodopa therapy remains the gold standard of symptomatic treatment for Parkinson's disease. However, long-term therapy with levodopa is less than satisfactory as disability continues to progress and most patients develop levodopa-associated motor fluctuations and dyskinesias within a few years of treatment. Many patients ultimately develop disability due to difficulty with balance or cognition. For this reason, much research in Parkinson's disease today focuses on how to forestall disability and maintain or improve function over the long-term.

What are the basic strategies used for the treatment of Parkinson's disease?

Treatment strategies are potentially divided into those that are:
a) symptomatic, **b)** neuroprotective, or **c)** restorative.

Symptomatic therapies are those that improve signs and symptoms without affecting the underlying disease state. Degeneration of the substantia nigra in Parkinson's disease causes a striatal dopamine deficiency. Administration of levodopa increases dopamine concentration in the striatum. Levodopa is administered in combination with a peripheral dopadecarboxylase inhibitor (DDCI) to minimize nausea and to facilitate appropriate resorption and to get adequate peak levels. Neuroprotection prevents neurons from undergoing cell death.

Catechol-O-methyltransferase (COMT) inhibitors further inhibit levodopa's peripheral metabolism, thereby extending the half-life and duration of action of each levodopa dose. Monoamine oxidase type B (MAO-B) inhibitors increase dopamine activity in the brain by inhibiting its metabolism. Dopamine agonists provide symptomatic benefit by directly stimulating post-synaptic striatal dopamine receptors. Other symptomatic medications used in the treatment of Parkinson's disease include amantadine, which augments dopamine release, and anticholinergics such as trihexyphenidyl and benztropine, which block striatal cholinergic function. Each of these medications is discussed in greater detail below.

Neuroprotective therapies are those that slow neuronal degeneration, thereby delaying disease progression. There are no proven neuroprotective therapies available for Parkinson's disease. New medications are currently being evaluated for their ability to slow disease progression.

Restorative therapies are those that aim to replace lost neurons. One approach to replacing lost neurons is the transplantation of cells. Transplanted cells have been demonstrated to survive, restore neuronal connections, and increase dopamine concentration. However, transplantation has not been demonstrated to provide benefit for patients. Stem cells, genetically engineered cells, and cells from other parts of the human body are being developed for transplantation and will be evaluated for possible restorative effects.

What is levodopa?

Levodopa is the chemical precursor of dopamine. The dopamine depletor reserpine was found to produce parkinsonian symptoms in rats in the late 1950s[2]. In addition, post-mortem examinations of Parkinson's disease patients revealed decreased dopamine concentration in the striatum, correlating with the loss of nigro-striatal neurons in the substantia nigra[3]. As dopamine does not cross the blood-brain barrier, its precursor, levodopa, was tested as dopamine replacement therapy. Levodopa was shown to dramatically improve parkinsonian symptoms[4].

The main difficulties with early levodopa therapy were insufficent response and a high incidence of nausea and vomiting. Concomitant administration of peripheral dopadecarboxylase inhibitors was found to improve the clinical utility of levodopa by reducing its peripheral breakdown[5]. Decreased peripheral dopamine production reduces the incidence of nausea and vomiting and allows more levodopa to cross the blood-brain barrier. The dopadecarboxylase inhibitors carbidopa and benserazide are most commonly combined with levodopa for this purpose.

What are the pharmacokinetics of levodopa?

Levodopa, or l-dihydroxyphenylalanine, is a large neutral amino acid. After oral ingestion, it is absorbed in the proximal small intestine by a saturable, carrier-mediated transport system. Absorption can be delayed by meals [6] and increased gastric acidity [7]. Absorbed levodopa is not bound to plasma protein and its half-life is approximately one hour [8]. To exert an anti-parkinsonian effect, levadopa must cross the blood-brain barrier by way of the large neutral amino acid carrier transport system.

What are the main advantages of levodopa?

Of all the available oral medications, levodopa provides the greatest improvement for motor features of PD. It extends life expectancy and there is no reliable evidence that it hastens loss of dopamine neurons [114, 115]. In addition, it has fewer short-term side effects than dopamine agonists including less somnolence, hallucinations and edema.

What is levodopa/carbidopa?

Levodopa/carbidopa (Sinemet®, Nacom®) is a combination of carbidopa, a peripheral dopadecarboxylase inhibitors, and levodopa. Carbidopa lessens the peripheral (blood) decarboxylation of levodopa, thereby decreasing the incidence of nausea and increasing the central (brain) availability of levodopa. The addition of carbidopa reduces the amount of levodopa needed by about 75% [9]. Approximately 75 to 100 mg of carbidopa are required to saturate peripheral dopadecarboxylase [5]. Nonetheless, some patients require carbidopa in doses up to 200 mg per day to reduce or eliminate nausea. The half-life of levodopa when administered with carbidopa is approximately 90 minutes [9]. Standard, or immediate release, levodopa/carbidopa can be taken with or without meals. When taken with or shortly after a meal, its absorption is mildly decreased and delayed.

Patients with early PD usually find that the levodopa benefit lasts from dose to dose (stable response) and these individuals will usually not notice any difference in benefit taking levodopa/carbidopa with or without a meal. If such a patient experiences nausea in association with levodopa/carbidopa intake, taking the medication just after a meal commonly helps reduce the nausea.

In contrast, patients with moderate or advanced disease who find that benefit from levodopa wears off prior to the next dose taking effect, will often find that the benefit is less and will not last as long if they take it with a meal. Therefore, levodopa/carbidopa is usually administered one half hour or more before, or one hour or more after meals to achieve the most consistent absorption and greatest clinical benefit.

Although levodopa competes with other large, neutral amino acids (proteins) for transport across the blood-brain barrier, ingestion of a meal will not noticeably diminish the levodopa response for most patients. However, patients with marked fluctuations are more dependent on continuous levodopa delivery to the brain and may be sensitive to the small changes in bioavailability that occur after eating a meal. Patients with fluctuations who find that meals interfere with the levodopa response may want to consider a low protein or protein redistributed diet.

Are generic forms of levodopa/carbidopa available and do they have the same effect?

Generic forms of levodopa/carbidopa are available. They may contain slightly less or slightly more levodopa. Most patients do not notice a difference between generic and brand formulations, however, 20-30% of patients, especially those with motor fluctuations may notice worsening of symptoms when changing to a generic formulation[10,11].

What is levodopa/benserazide?

Levodopa/benserazide (Madopar®) is a combination of benserazide, a peripheral dopadecarboxylase inhibitors, and levodopa. It is used similarly to levodopa/carbidopa. This preparation is available outside the United States.

How do I initiate standard levodopa/carbidopa?

A commonly used initial target dose is carbidopa/levodopa 25/100 three times a day (TID), starting with half of a 25/100 tablet each day for the first week and increasing by a half tablet per day each week until the target dose is reached. The final dose must be tailored to the individual patient response. If there is a need to improve symptoms more quickly, the dose can potentially be increased by half of a 25/100 tablet every two to three days. The "start low" and "go slow" regimen helps avoid side effects such as nausea. The initial target dose of carbidopa/levodopa 25/100 TID is based more on convention than scientific evidence. Further research is necessary to determine the optimal initial target dose and interdose interval.

What are the side effects of levodopa/carbidopa and levodopa/benserazide?

The most common side effect of levodopa/carbidopa and levodopa/ benserazide is nausea. This is due to stimulation of the vomiting center in the medulla by dopamine formed in the bloodstream. If a patient has difficulty initiating the medication due to nausea, they should try taking it with a carbohydrate snack or immediately following a meal. Additional carbidopa (Lodosyn®, which is not available outside the US) may be prescribed. These steps will allow the vast majority of patients to tolerate levodopa medications without much difficulty. Where available, the use of a peripherally acting dopamine blocking drug, such as domperidone (Motilium®) is very helpful to alleviate refractory nausea.

Other potential side effects include orthostatic hypotension (lightheadedness), confusion, hallucinations, delusions, and sleepiness. Orthostatic hypotension can usually be countered with medications such as midodrine (Proamatine®) or fludrocortisone (Florinef®) [12]. Cognitive side effects typically occur later in the disease in patients who have developed underlying dementia. Confusion may occasionally improve with a decrease in levodopa dose. Hallucinations and delusions can be treated with atypical neuroleptics that have minimal parkinsonian side effects (see below).

What is levodopa/carbidopa Controlled Release (CR)?

Levodopa/carbidopa CR (Sinemet CR®) is a controlled-release preparation. It is more slowly absorbed and provides more sustained serum levels than standard levodopa/carbidopa [13]. It is best absorbed when taken with food and levodopa bioavailability is about 75-80% that of standard levodopa/carbidopa [14]. One potential drawback is that it takes about a half an hour longer to begin to exert its effect. This has no noticeable effect in early PD, but patients with more advanced disease may notice a delayed kick in. The initial target dose is carbidopa/levodopa CR 25/100 TID or 50/200 BID, usually starting with 100 mg levodopa per day and slowly increasing over a period of a few weeks. To convert a patient from standard levodopa/carbidopa to levodopa/carbidopa CR, the daily dosage is increased by approximately 20-25% while the number of daily doses is decreased by 30-50% [15,16].

Patients with moderate or advanced disease who experience a delayed kick in of effect on levodopa/carbidopa CR often need a small amount of standard levodopa/carbidopa as part of the first morning dose to act as a "booster" and bring on symptomatic benefit more quickly. This is often accomplished by adding one carbidopa/levodopa 25/100 tablet to the first CR dose of the day. Patients on standard carbidopa/levodopa who need a bedtime dose often use the CR formulation for that dose so that benefit into the night will be more prolonged.

What is levodopa/benserazide HBS?

Levodopa/benserazide hydrodynamically balanced system (Madopar HBS®, Madopar depot®) is an extended- release levodopa preparation available outside the U.S, containing hydrocolloids, fats, and the decarboxylase inhibitor benserazide. Levodopa/benserazide HBS "floats" on stomach contents for five to twelve hours allowing levodopa to be slowly absorbed. Compared to standard levodopa/benserazide, levodopa bioavailability is about 60%, so a switch usually necessitates a dosage increase [22]. As with other extended-release levodopa preparations, it is often supplemented with a small dose of standard formulation levodopa to provide an early morning "kick".

What are the side effects of levodopa/carbidopa CR?

Side effects of levodopa/carbidopa CR are similar to those of standard levodopa/carbidopa. However, because levodopa/carbidopa CR persists longer in the blood, acute transient side effects may also persist longer with levodopa/carbidopa CR. For example, a patient who experiences nausea or lightheadedness for half an hour after taking standard levodopa/carbidopa may have those side effects for an hour after taking levodopa/carbidopa CR. However, when given the same mg strength CR vs. standard tablets, some patients will find that such symptoms are diminished on the CR formulation because of its lower bioavailability.

What is Parcopa?

Parcopa® is levodopa/carbidopa in an orally disintegrating tablet that dissolves on the tongue. It dissolves within seconds, and then levodopa/carbidopa is carried in the saliva past the stomach, into the proximal small bowel where it is absorbed. It was approved based on demonstrations of bioequivalence with standard levodopa/carbidopa.

Parcopa is available in three strengths: carbidopa/levodopa 25/100, 10/100, and 25/250. Parcopa should be removed from its package with dry hands, placed on the tongue, and allowed to dissolve. It can be taken with or without water, and can be stored in pill bottles and carried and cut like standard levodopa/carbidopa. Tablets of different strengths can be taken together. Patients can use Parcopa as their main source of levodopa or substitute for standard levodopa/carbidopa tablets when desired.

The main advantage of Parcopa is the convenience afforded by being able to take it without water. It can be kept be kept by the bed and easily taken overnight or in the morning without getting up for water. Similarly, it is convenient to take while travelling. Some patients report that the onset of benefit with Parcopa is quicker than with standard levodopa/carbidopa but this has not yet been rigorously studied.

Parcopa has the same side effects as standard levodopa/carbidopa.
In addition, patients should be instructed that occasionally, a dark color (red, brown, or black) may appear in saliva, sweat, or urine. This discoloration is clinically insignificant.

What is levodopa/carbidopa/entacapone?

Levodopa/carbidopa/entacapone (Stalevo®) is a combination of standard levodopa/carbidopa plus entacapone in a single tablet. It was approved based on demonstrations of bioequivalence with standard levodopa/carbidopa plus entacapone administered as separate tablets.

Entacapone (Comtan®, Comtess®) is a peripherally acting catechol-O-methyltransferase (COMT) inhibitor. COMT is one of the main enzymes responsible for levodopa's metabolism and clearance from the blood. The addition of entacapone to standard levodopa/carbidopa prolongs the levodopa half-life to approximately 2.25 hours [9]. This provides more sustained levels of levodopa in the blood.

In patients with wearing-off motor fluctuations, switching from levodopa/carbidopa to levodopa/carbidopa/entacapone reduces OFF time and helps smooth the clinical response. Levodopa/carbidopa/entacapone provides as quick an onset of action as standard levodopa/carbidopa but lasts longer and smooths levodopa plasma levels

Parkinson's Disease

resulting in less pulsatile and more continuous delivery of levodopa. Based on preclinical studies, there is interest in the potential benefit of using levodopa/carbidopa/entacapone as the initial levodopa preparation as discussed below.

An open label study was performed to evaluate Stalevo compared with immediate-release levodopa/carbidopa plus entacapone in PD patients with end-of-dose wearing-off[17]. As expected, there was no difference in motor improvement or side effects. Patients on Stalevo were then switched to an equivalent dose of levodopa/carbidopa and separate entacapone for an additional two-week period. Patients reported significantly better quality of life with Stalevo (p < 0.001) and 81% indicated that they preferred treatment with Stalevo over separate tablets.

Stalevo is available as 50, 100, and 150 mg tablets with this designation indication the mg dosage of levodopa in the tablet. Each tablet also contains carbidopa in a 1:4 ratio with levodopa, plus 200 mg of entacapone. When used as initial levodopa therapy, Stalevo can be initiated at a dosage of one 50/12.5/200 mg tablet (Stalevo 50) BID for one week and then increased to Stalevo 50 QID. Further escalation can be undertaken as clinically necessary. Side effects are the same as those caused by levodopa/carbidopa and entacapone and potentially include increased dyskinesia, nausea and diarrhea. Patients who are receiving standard levodopa/carbidopa and entacapone as separate tablets can be switched to the equivalent dose Stalevo for increased convenience and to help assure correct dosing of entacapone.

For patients with end of dose wearing-off, switching from standard levodopa/carbidopa to Stalevo is analogous to adding entacapone, which reduces OFF time, and improves PD symptoms. It is recommended that patients taking less than 600 mg/day (US) or 800 mg/day (EU) levodopa and not experiencing dyskinesia can be directly switched to the levodopa equivalent dose Stalevo. Patients with dyskinesia and those taking more than 600-800 mg/day levodopa are more likely to experience emergence or worsening of dyskinesia and may therefore require a downward titration of levodopa[19]. For these patients it is recommended that entacapone first be added and then levodopa titrated as necessary. Once the patient is stabilized on levodopa/carbidopa plus entacapone, they can be switched to the equivalent dose Stalevo. When switching a patient from levodopa/DDCI to Stalevo, it is usually recommended that levodopa/DDCI is discontinued the previous night and Stalevo is started the next morning.

When I begin levodopa should I use standard levodopa/carbidopa, levodopa/carbidopa CR, or levodopa/carbidopa/entacapone?

Standard levodopa/carbidopa, levodopa/carbidopa CR, and levodopa/carbidopa/entacapone are equally effective in improving motor symptoms when levodopa is first required. Generic formulations of standard and CR levodopa/carbidopa are available and are less expensive than the brand formulations. Patients find the levodopa/carbidopa CR or levodopa/carbidopa/entacapone more convenient because fewer daily doses may be required.

There is interest as to whether more continuous dopamine receptor stimulation as afforded by levodopa/carbidopa CR or levodopa/carbidopa/entacapone can forestall the development of long-term complications including motor fluctuations and dyskinesia. A five-year study comparing standard and CR levodopa/carbidopa found no difference in the incidence of fluctuations and dyskinesia [20]. However, levodopa/carbidopa CR was administered on a BID schedule in this study and that may be too infrequent to provide sufficiently continuous stimulation. Levodopa/carbidopa/entacapone administered on a QID schedule to MPTP monkeys caused less motor fluctuations and dyskinesia than the same daily levodopa/ carbidopa dose administered QID without entacapone or BID with or without entacapone [21].

A clinical trial (STRIDE-PD) is now underway with patients randomized to treatment with levodopa/carbidopa or Stalevo when levodopa is first required to determine if Stalevo will delay the onset of dyskinesia compared to standard levodopa/carbidopa. Another clinical trial, the FIRST-STEP study, will evaluate whether Stalevo provides greater symptom benefit than levodopa/carbidopa at the same levodopa dose when used as initial levodopa therapy in PD.

Once patients develop troublesome motor fluctuations and dyskinesia, levodopa/carbidopa CR becomes more problematic because of variability in its absorption. Standard levodopa formulations (levodopa/carbidopa and levodopa/carbidopa/entacapone) provide a more consistent response.

What symptoms of Parkinson's disease are best alleviated by levodopa therapy?

Levodopa therapy is the cornerstone of symptomatic treatment. It is most effective in relieving bradykinesia and rigidity, while its effect on tremor is

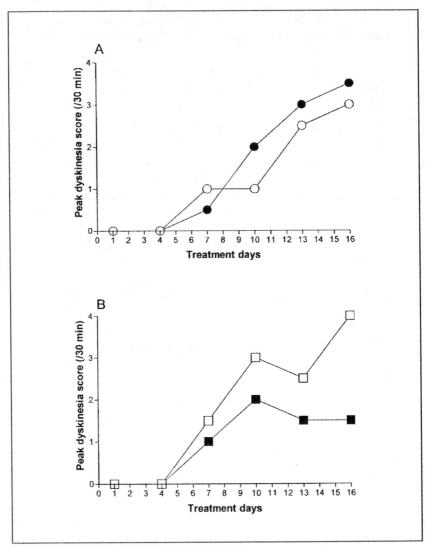

Figure 6.0. *Peak dyskinesia scores in MPTP-treated common marmosets on day 16 of administration of L-dopa (12.5 mg/kg + carbidopa 12.5 mg/kg p.o.) b.i.d. (**A**, open circles) and L-dopa (12.5 mg/kg + carbidopa 12.5 mg/kg p.o.) b.i.d. plus entacapone (12.5 mng/kg p.o.) b.i.d. (**A**, filled circles) or L-dopa (6.25 mg/kg + carbidopa 12.5 mg/kg p.o.) q.i.d. (**B**, open squares) and L-dopa (6.25 mg/kg + carbidopa 12.5 mg/kg p.o.) q.i.d. plus entacapone (12.5 mg/kg p.o.) q.i.d. (**B**, filled squares). Data are median score on each day (n = 4 per group)[21].*

highly variable[22]. Symptoms such as balance impairment and dementia are not alleviated by levodopa. Depression, freezing, autonomic nervous system dysfunction, and pain are sometimes helped by levodopa. When assessing the

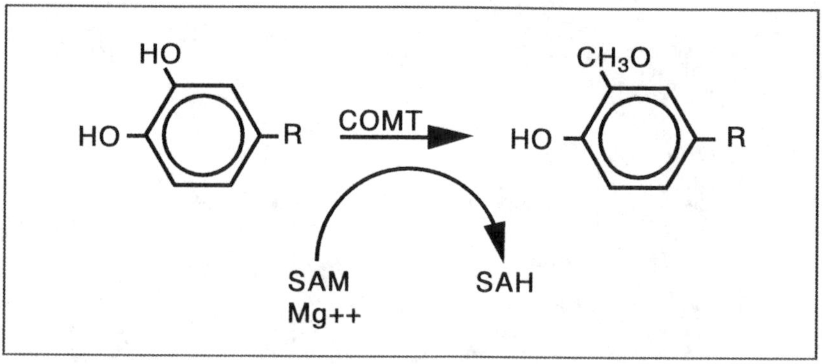

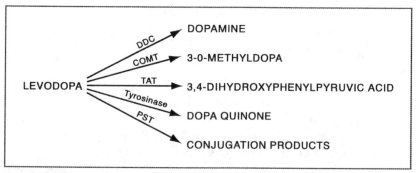

Figure 6.1. *Methylation of catechol substrate by COMT.*
SAM = S-adenosyl-L-methionine; SAH = S-adenosyl-L-homocysteine; R = side chain.

Figure 6.2. *The metabolism of levodopa.*
DDC = dopa decarboxylase; COMT = catechol-O-methyltransferase;
TAT = tyrosine aminotransferase; PST = phenol sulphotransferase.

benefit of levodopa, one should evaluate motor function, specifically bradykinesia and rigidity. Symptomatic improvement may or may not occur if a patient only has tremor. In addition, improvement may be difficult to detect if symptoms are minimal. Improvement with levodopa therapy is usually apparent with more advanced disease as motor dysfunction, bradykinesia, and rigidity become more obvious.

What are COMT inhibitors?

Catechol-O-methyltransferase (COMT) is one of the main enzymes responsible for the metabolism of levodopa, dopamine, other catecholamines (adrenaline and noradrenaline), and their metabolites. COMT catalyzes the transfer of a methyl group from S-adenosyl-L-methionine (SAM) to the hydroxyl group of catecholamines (figure 6.1)[23].

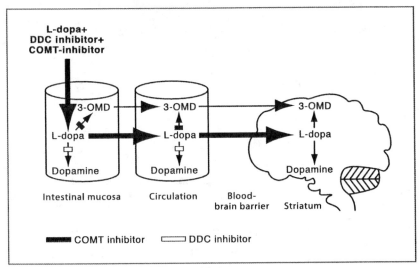

Figure 6.3. *Mechanism of peripheral COMT inhibition.*

COMT is widely distributed throughout the body [24,25] including central nervous system neurons and glia, but not nigrostriatal dopamine neurons [26]. Levodopa is metabolized by several different enzymes (figure 6.2), with dopa decarboxylase and COMT being most important. When levodopa is administered with a peripheral dopa decarboxylase inhibitor such as carbidopa or benserazide, COMT metabolism of levodopa predominates. COMT metabolizes levodopa to 3-O-methyldopa (3-OMD). 3-OMD has the potential to decrease levodopa absorption and efficacy [27,28], although at the concentrations present in PD patients, this does not appear to be an important consideration.

Peripherally acting COMT inhibitors block COMT in the gut and periphery. By decreasing levodopa metabolism, they make more levodopa available for transport across the blood-brain barrier over a longer time and also reduce 3-OMD production (figure 6.3) [29]. When COMT inhibitors are added to levodopa therapy, striatal dopamine concentrations increase [29]. Central COMT inhibition might further increase striatal dopamine concentration by inhibiting the metabolism of dopamine to homovanillic acid (HVA) [29].

What is entacapone?

Entacapone (Comtan®, Comtess®) is a reversible peripheral COMT inhibitor (figure 6.4) [30]. Its half-life is approximately half-an-hour (0.4-0.7 hrs) [31]. Entacapone is usually administered at a dose of 200 mg with each levodopa dose, up to a usual

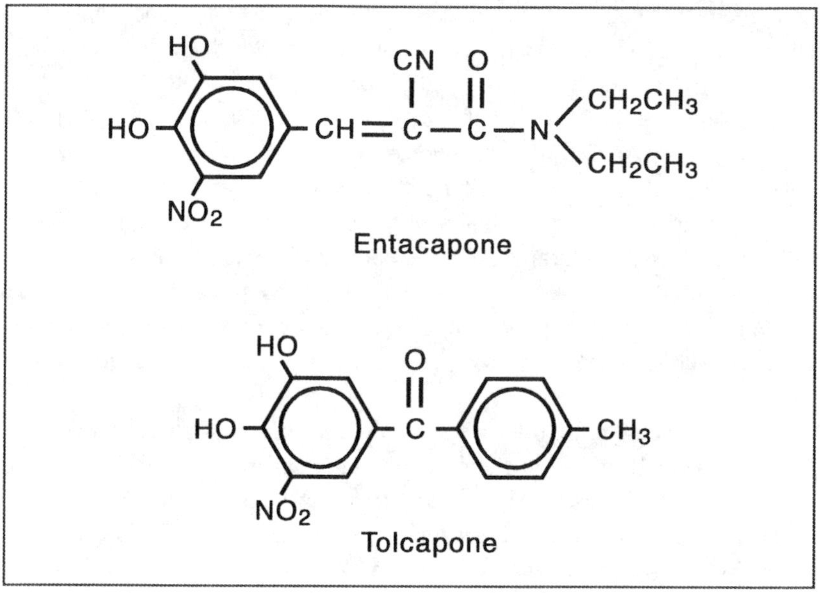

Figure 6.4. *The structures of entacapone and tolcapone.*

maximum of eight times a day (1600 mg) in the US and ten times a day (2000 mg) in the EU. Entacapone reduces the peripheral metabolism of levodopa to 3-OMD [31], prolongs the levodopa half-life from 1.3 to 2.4 hours and increases levodopa bioavailability (area under the curve) by approximately 35% [32]. side effects are mostly those related to increased dopaminergic stimulation. Dyskinesia may emerge or worsen when entacapone is added, and some patients may require a reduction in levodopa dose, usually on the order of 10-25%.

Those patients likely to require a reduction in levodopa dose are those who have moderate or severe dyskinesia on levodopa alone and to a lesser extent, those on more than 600-800 mg levodopa/day. Other dopaminergic side effects include nausea and hallucinations. These side effects can usually be reduced or eliminated by decreasing the levodopa dose. Approximately 10% of patients experience diarrhea and 2% discontinue entacapone because of this side effect. Onset of diarrhea typically occurs within 4-12 weeks but may be earlier or later.
The mechanism of this side effect is unknown. Patients should be informed that they might notice a brownish orange discoloration of the urine or sweat that is not clinically relevant. There is no known hepatotoxicity associated with entacapone and there is no requirement for liver function test monitoring. In clinical trials, elevations of liver function tests were no more common in entacapone-treated patients than placebo-treated patients.

Entacapone is effective in reducing OFF time, improving motor function, and allowing levodopa dose reductions in patients with motor fluctuations on levodopa. The Parkinson Study Group (PSG) conducted a multi-center, double-blind, placebo-controlled trial of entacapone in 205 fluctuating PD patients over a 24-week period [33]. This trial is known as SEESAW (Safety and Efficacy of Entacapone Study Assessing Wearing-Off). Patients were randomized to receive either entacapone 200 mg or placebo with each levodopa dose. OFF time was reduced by 17.6% in entacapone-treated patients compared to 4.5% in placebo-treated patients ($p < 0.01$). The total daily levodopa dose was decreased by 11.6% in the entacapone group compared to an increase of 2.5% in the placebo group ($p < 0.001$). UPDRS ADL, motor, and total scores all improved significantly.

A similar study design was used in the NOMECOMT (Nordic Multicenter Entacapone COMT) trial [34]. In entacapone-treated patients, mean OFF time decreased by 22% ($p < 0.001$) and mean ON time increased by more than 13% ($p < 0.01$). UPDRS scores improved significantly and daily levodopa dose and intake frequency were significantly reduced.

In an open-label extension of the NOMECOMT study, called NOMESAFE, 92% of patients maintained benefit regarding OFF time through three years. At three years, when entacapone was withdrawn symptoms worsened, demonstrating that entacapone was still providing benefit [35].

The Celomen study was a double-blind, randomized trial that evaluated the efficacy and safety of entacapone in PD patients [36]. Three hundred and one PD patients (the majority with motor fluctuations) were randomized to receive entacapone or placebo with each dose of standard or controlled-release (CR) levodopa, and were followed for 24 weeks. Significant improvements were observed in UPDRS activities of daily living and motor scores in patients taking entacapone ($p < 0.05$). ON time also increased by a mean of 1.7 hours while OFF time decreased by 1.5 hours compared to placebo ($p < 0.05$). There was a decrease in the daily levodopa dose of 54 mg in patients taking entacapone, compared to an increase of 27 mg in the placebo group ($p < 0.05$). The efficacy of entacapone was comparable between patients using standard and CR levodopa preparations. Eight percent of patients taking entacapone experienced diarrhea compared to 4% of patients taking placebo, and was rarely severe.

Another large open-label multi-center study of patients with end-of-dose wearing-off also found that the addition of entacapone was associated with improvement in patient quality of life as measured by improvement in the eight-item Parkinson's Disease Questionnaire (PDQ-8)[37]. Investigators' Clinical Global Impression of Change (CGI-C) revealed that 76.5% of patients treated with entacapone showed improvement in global status after 4 weeks of therapy.

Entacapone also enhances the clinical efficacy of controlled release levodopa/carbidopa[38]. One study found that the addition of entacapone to levodopa prolonged the ON phase by 37%. ON time correlated with a significant increase in levodopa bioavailability (AUC).

Athough entacapone is approved as an adjunct to levodopa for the treatment of PD patients with end-of-dose wearing-off, a multi-center, double-blind study found that entacapone also improved a variety of quality-of-life measures in PD patients who were not experiencing motor fluctuations[39]. Treatment with entacapone resulted in significant improvement in several quality-of-life measures, including the Parkinson Disease Questionnaire 39 (PDQ-39), the 36-item Short-Form Health Survey, the Parkinson's Symptom Inventory, and investigator and subject Clinical Global Assessments. However, the addition of entacapone did not improve UPDRS motor scores in this group of patients who were not experiencing motor fluctuations.

There is evidence that pulsatile stimulation of dopamine receptors may contribute to dyskinesia. The continuous dopamine stimulation hypothesis suggests that the use of levodopa in conjunction with a COMT inhibitor to extend its half-life and reduce levodopa fluctuations may reduce the risk of developing motor complications[40]. In a preclinical animal model study, the addition of entacapone to a levodopa QID regimen resulted in less dyskinesia than the same levodopa regimen without entacapone[41]. This study suggests that the use of entacapone when levodopa is first introduced may result in more continuous delivery of levodopa and reduce the risk of motor complications compared to levodopa/carbidopa.

The STRIDE-PD (STalevo Reduction in Dyskinesia Evaluation) will evaluate whether the use of levodopa/carbidopa/entacapone (Stalevo) results in a delay to the onset of dyskinesia compared to levodopa/carbidopa.

What is tolcapone?

Tolcapone (Tasmar®) is a reversible COMT inhibitor (figure 6.4). It has the capacity to induce fatal hepatic failure and strict liver function test monitoring is required. Because of this risk, its use is reserved for patients with motor fluctuations on levodopa who do not respond to or who could not tolerate other adjunctive therapies. If substantial clinical benefits are not seen within three weeks of initiation of treatment, tolcapone should be discontinued. Animal studies indicate that tolcapone exerts central as well as peripheral COMT inhibition [42]. It is rapidly absorbed and has a half-life of approximately two hours [43]. It is introduced at a dose of 100 mg TID and this is the usual maintenance dose. The dose can be increased to 200 mg TID in selected patients in whom the additional benefit is felt to outweigh the additional risk. Other side effects are mostly those related to increased dopaminergic stimulation [44].

Patients with levodopa-induced dyskinesia often have an initial rapid increase in dyskinesia necessitating a 25-50% reduction in levodopa dose. Alternatively, the levodopa dose can be reduced by 25-50% at the time tolcapone is initiated and then titrated further as appropriate. Additional dopaminergic side effects include nausea and hallucinations. These side effects can usually be reduced or eliminated by decreasing the levodopa dose. Approximately 10% of patients experience diarrhea and 3% discontinue tolcapone because of this side effect. Onset of diarrhea is usually delayed for four to twelve weeks after initiation of therapy but uncommon after six months [44].

Tolcapone improves motor function and allows levodopa dose reductions in patients on levodopa therapy with either motor fluctuations or a stable response. Two studies evaluated the efficacy of adding tolcapone to levodopa therapy in patients experiencing motor fluctuations [45,46]. OFF time was reduced by two hours per day in patients taking 100 mg TID and 2.5 hours per day in patients taking 200 mg TID [46].

In a double-blind, placebo-controlled study evaluating tolcapone in 298 patients on levodopa without motor fluctuations, tolcapone produced significant reductions in activities of daily living and motor function at both 100 mg TID and 200 mg TID dosing. These improvements were maintained for up to 12 months [44]. However, tolcapone is not indicated for use in patients without motor fluctuations because the benefit does not appear to justify the risk.

Does tolcapone cause liver damage?

In clinical trials, hepatic enzymes alanine aminotransferase (ALT) and aspartate aminotransferase (AST), were elevated to more than three times the upper limits of normal in approximately 1% and 3% of patients treated with tolcapone 100 mg TID and 200 mg TID, respectively. Increases to more than eight times the upper limits of normal occurred in 0.3% and 0.7% of patients. Women were more likely than men to experience an increase in hepatic enzymes (approximately 5% versus 2%). Elevations usually occurred within six weeks to six months of starting treatment. When tolcapone was discontinued, enzymes generally returned to normal within two to three weeks, but in some cases took as long as one to two months. None of the patients in clinical trials developed clinical sequelae of liver injury.

Tolcapone became available for clinical use in August 1997 in Europe and February 1998 in the U.S. By October 1998, three cases of fatal hepatic failure were identified from approximately sixty thousand patients on tolcapone, providing approximately forty thousand patient-years of worldwide use [47]. This incidence was approximately 10-100 times higher than the background incidence of fatal hepatic failure in the general population. All three patients were women in their seventies who were placed on tolcapone but did not undergo liver function monitoring. Time from initiation of tolcapone to clinical illness ranged form eight to twelve weeks. Recognition of the potential for life-threatening hepatocellular injury prompted the withdrawal of tolcapone in Europe, and in the U.S. the FDA revised the labeling. This labeling change emphasized the need for rigorous liver function enzyme monitoring.

The risks of tolcapone use should be reviewed with the patient and the patient should provide written informed consent. ALT/AST levels should be obtained at baseline, every two weeks for the first year of therapy, every four weeks for the next six months, and then every eight weeks for the duration of administration. Tolcapone should be discontinued if ALT/AST exceeds the upper limit of normal. If meaningful clinical benefit is not observed within three weeks, tolcapone should be discontinued.

What are dopamine agonists?

Dopamine agonists directly stimulate post-synaptic dopamine receptors and unlike levodopa they do not require enzymatic conversion [48]. They provide symptomatic benefit as monotherapy in early disease and as adjuncts to levodopa in later disease.

What are the side effects of dopamine agonists?

Dopamine agonists can cause nausea, vomiting, and orthostatic hypotension by stimulating peripheral dopamine receptors. They may also cause central

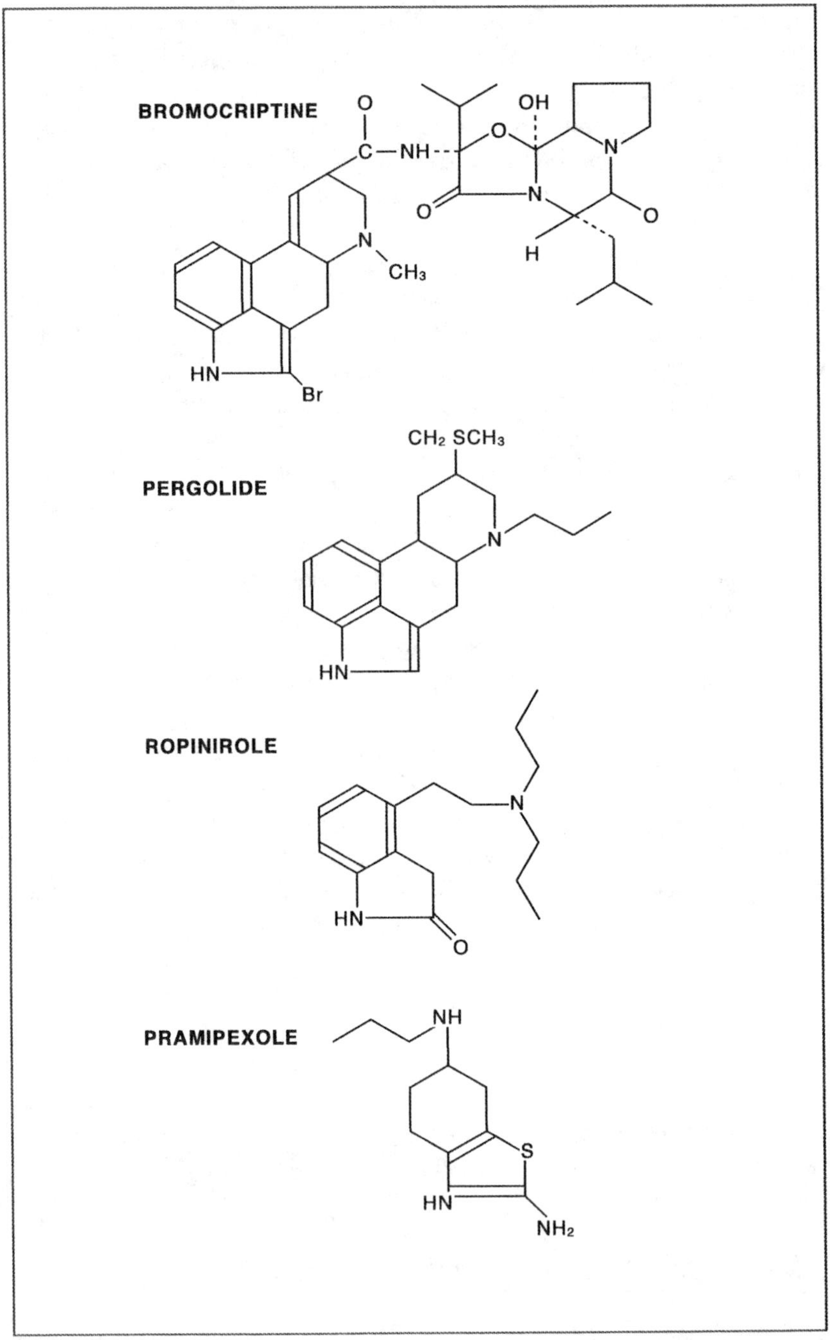

Figure 6.5. *Chemical structures of bromocriptine and pergolide, ropinirole and pramipexole.*

dopaminergic side effects such as nightmares, hallucinations, or daytime sleepiness. Cognitive side effects are dose related but nausea and orthostatic hypotension can occur even with small initial doses. Other possible side effects include leg edema and constipation [49].

Should dopamine agonists be given with or without food?

Meals have little effect on the extent of absorption of dopamine agonists and they can be taken with or without food. Patients with nausea should take their medication after a meal. For patients on combination therapy with levodopa, the dopamine agonist is usually scheduled to be taken with levodopa as a matter of convenience.

What is bromocriptine?

Bromocriptine (Parlodel®) is an ergot alkaloid dopamine receptor agonist (figure 6.5). It is a strong D2 receptor agonist and a weak D1 receptor antagonist (figure 6.6). It stimulates both pre- and post-synaptic receptors, and its half-life is approximately seven hours [9]. It can be initiated at a dose of one half of a 2.5 mg tablet per day, and increased every third day by 2.5 mg to a daily dose in the range of 10-40 mg [49]. A TID dosing schedule is typically used. Potential side effects include nausea, vomiting, orthostatic hypotension, confusion, hallucinations, anorexia, and erythromelalgia, a painful, reddish discoloration of the skin. Retroperitoneal fibrosis has been reported in a few patients who received long-term therapy at high dosages.

| | Receptor Binding | | | | | |
	D_2	D_3	D_1	$5HT_{1/2}$	α_1	α_2
Bromocriptine[1]	++	+	+	++	++	++
Pergolide[2]	++	++	++	++	+	++
Ropinirole	++	+++	-	-	-	-
Pramipexole	++	+++	-	-	-	-

[1] Bromocriptine is a D_1 Antagonist   [2] Pergolide is a D_1 Agonist

Figure 6.6. *Receptor binding of bromocriptine, pergolide, ropinirole and pramipexole.*

What is pergolide?

Pergolide (Permax®) is a semisynthetic, clavine ergot derivative dopamine agonist (figure 6.5). In contrast to bromocriptine, it is a strong D2 receptor agonist and a weak D1 receptor agonist (figure 6.6). Peak plasma levels are achieved in one to two hours, and its half-life is approximately 20-27 hours[9]. The starting dose is 0.05 mg tablet per day, with an initial target dose of 0.25 mg TID achieved over four to six weeks. The usual maximum recommended dose is 4-5 mg per day in divided doses. Potential side effects include nausea, vomiting, orthostatic hypotension, cognitive dysfunction, increased liver enzymes, erythromelalgia, and peripheral edema[50]. Valvular heart disease can also occur[51].

Pergolide was compared to placebo as an adjunct to levodopa in patients with motor fluctuations[52]. Pergolide permitted a mean levodopa dose reduction of 24.7% compared with 4.9% in the placebo group (p < .001). Motor function improved by 35% in pergolide-treated patients compared with 17% in placebo-treated patients (p < .001) and OFF time decreased by 32% compared with 4% (p < .001). Although new onset or worsening of dyskinesia was observed in 62% of the pergolide group compared to 25% of the placebo group, dyskinesia was generally controlled by a reduction of levodopa dose such that there was no difference in dyskinesia disability by the end of the study.

The PELMOPET study (pergolide-versus-L-dopa-monotherapy-and-positron-emission-tomography trial) was a multi-center, double-blind, three-year trial that compared pergolide monotherapy (n = 148) with levodopa monotherapy (n = 146) in early levodopa-naïve PD patients[53]. The severity of motor complications was significantly lower and the time to dyskinesia onset was significantly delayed in the patients who received pergolide (3.23 mg/day) compared with those who received levodopa (504 mg/day). However, the time to onset of motor complications was not longer in patients who received pergolide after three years. In addition, there was significantly greater symptomatic benefit in motor symptoms in patients who received levodopa. Side effects caused 17.6% of pergolide patients and 9.6% of levodopa patients to discontinue therapy.

Retrospective studies and case reports point towards a higher frequency of valvular heart disease in patients taking pergolide, but further prospective studies are necessary to establish the true prevalence and incidence of this problem[54,55]. It has been suggested that activation of 5-HT2B receptors may be the basis for this observation[56]. Pergolide-induced valvulopathy appears to be rare, but it seems prudent to obtain an echocardiogram of the heart intermittently in patients chronically treated with pergolide.

Sleepiness is also common in dopamine agonists as a class, and one study found that treatment with pergolide 1 mg at bedtime resulted in worsened actigraphic measures of sleep efficiency and sleep fragmentation compared to patients who received placebo [57].

What is ropinirole?

Ropinirole (Requip®) is a highly selective D2 agonist with little affinity for D1, 5HT, muscarinic, or adrenergic receptors (figure 6.6). It is a non-ergoline dopamine agonist and has a half-life of approximately six hours (figure 6.5). Maximal plasma concentration is reached approximately 1.5 hours after administration in fasted patients and approximately four hours when taken with meals [58]. The starting dose is 0.25 mg TID, with an initial target dose of 3 mg TID achieved over eight weeks. Further escalation should be undertaken as clinically necessary with a recommended maximum dose of 24 mg per day. Side effects are similar to other dopamine agonists and include nausea, somnolence, insomnia, dizziness, dyspepsia, and headache [9].

Ropinirole is effective both as early monotherapy and as an adjunct to treatment with levodopa. A number of studies have demonstrated the safety and efficacy of ropinirole in the treatment of Parkinson's disease. One study compared ropinirole to placebo as add-on therapy in patients not optimally controlled on levodopa. At six months, 27.7% of ropinirole- treated patients had at least a 20% reduction in levodopa dose and at least a 20% reduction in OFF time compared with 11% in the placebo group (odds ratio = 4.4; 95% confidence interval, 1.53 to 12.66) [59]. Mean reduction of levodopa dose in the ropinirole group was 19.4%.

In a study of ropinirole as monotherapy in early stage patients, motor function was improved by 24% at six months in ropinirole-treated patients compared with a 3% worsening in placebo-treated patients (p < .001) (60. Significantly fewer ropinirole-treated patients required levodopa compared with placebo-treated patients (11% vs. 29%, p < 0.001). In a six-month study comparing ropinirole with levodopa in early stage patients, a similar percentage of patients in each group experienced greater than 30% improvement (48% vs. 58%), although levodopa-treated patients experienced significantly greater improvement overall (32% vs. 44%) [61].

Ropinirole has been demonstrated to reduce the incidence of dyskinesia when used in early PD [62]. In a five-year study, 268 de-novo PD patients were randomized to receive levodopa or ropinirole to which levodopa could be added if necessary.

At the completion of the study, patients in both groups had experienced benefit in parkinsonian symptoms, however, the benefit was significantly greater for those in the levodopa group compared to the ropinirole group (p < 0.008). On the other hand, dyskinesia had developed in only 20% of patients in the ropinirole group compared to 45% in the levodopa group (p < 0.001). Patients in the ropinirole group also developed significantly less disabling dyskinesia. Adverse effects such as hallucinations, somnolence and peripheral edema were more common in the ropinirole group. This study indicates that the strategy of starting symptomatic therapy with ropinirole and then adding levodopa later when necessary leads to less dyskinesia [62].

Does ropinirole slow the progression of PD?

One way to assess PD progression is by neuroimaging. 18F-dopa PET scans evaluate the amount of dopa that is taken up by remaining dopamine neurons and serves as an index of the number of remaining dopamine neurons. β-CIT SPECT scans evaluate the amount of β-CIT that binds to dopamine reuptake sites on dopamine neuron terminals and also serves as an index of the number of remaining dopamine neurons.

The REAL-PET [63] study was a two-year, double-blind, multinational study of 186 PD patients with no previous dopaminergic treatment. Patients were randomized to treatment with either levodopa or ropinirole to which open label levodopa could be added if necessary. The primary endpoint was the change in putamen 18F-dopa uptake on positron emission tomography (PET). There were 68 (74%) patients who completed the ropinirole arm and 69 (76%) who completed the levodopa arm. The change in 18F-dopa uptake at the end of the study compared to baseline was -13% for the ropinirole arm and -20% for the levodopa arm.

This is a relative difference of 35%, suggesting a slower disease progression with ropinirole compared to levodopa. However, direct pharmacologic effects of these medications, or compensatory mechanisms induced by them, cannot be excluded as possible alternative explanations for these results. Three percent of patients on ropinirole versus 27% on levodopa developed dyskinesia, however, patients on levodopa had significantly greater motor improvement.

What is pramipexole?

Pramipexole (Mirapex®) is a non-ergot D2/D3 agonist (figure 6-6). It is a synthetic amino-benzathiazol derivative that binds to D3 receptors with 7-fold greater affinity than to D2 or D4 receptors and has little affinity for D1, 5HT, muscarinic, or adrenergic receptors[64]. Pramipexole is introduced at a dose of 0.125 mg TID for one week and escalated over three weeks to an initial target dose of 0.5 mg TID. The usual recommended maximum dose is 4.5 mg/day. Side effects are similar to other dopamine agonists and include somnolence, nausea, constipation, insomnia, and hallucinations[65,66].

Pramipexole is effective both as early monotherapy and as an adjunct to treatment with levodopa. In a comparison of pramipexole to placebo as monotherapy in early disease, pramipexole significantly improved motor function and activities of daily living[65]. In a six-month trial comparing pramipexole to placebo as add-on therapy in patients with motor fluctuations on levodopa, OFF time was reduced by 17% in pramipexole-treated patients compared with 8% in placebo-treated patients (p < .01)[66]. Levodopa was reduced by 25% in the pramipexole group compared with 6% in the placebo group (p < .01). An open-label extension found that pramipexole demonstrated continued efficacy as an adjunct to levodopa for up to three years. After three years there was a gradual return to baseline motor disability consistent with disease progression. Common side effects in this long-term study included dyskinesia, dizziness, insomnia and hallucinations[67].

Pramipexole has been demonstrated to reduce the incidence of dyskinesia and motor fluctuations when used in early PD[68]. In the CALM-PD study, 301 patients with early PD who required dopaminergic therapy were randomized to receive either pramipexole or levodopa to which levodopa could be added if necessary. At the conclusion of the study, patients assigned to levodopa had greater improvement in motor function compared to pramipexole. However, 28% of patients on pramipexole developed wearing-off, dyskinesia or on-off motor fluctuations compared to 51% on levodopa. Although the overall incidence of dyskinesia was lower in the pramipexole group, when it came to disabling dyskinesia, they were both uncommon and not statistically different between levodopa and pramipexole after four years on treatment. Somnolence, hallucinations and peripheral edema were more common in the pramipexole group than the levodopa group.

This result is similar to the ropinirole vs. levodopa study. Both studies indicate that initial treatment with a dopamine agonist to which levodopa can be added leads to less motor fluctuations and dyskinesias than levodopa alone. These results are consistent with the Continuous Dopaminergic Stimulation hypothesis.

Does pramipexole slow the progression of PD?

The ability of pramipexole to slow disease progression was evaluated using -CIT SPECT scanning as an index of remaining dopamine neurons in the CALM-PD-CIT study [69]. This study included a subset of patients from the CALM-PD study. Eighty-two patients underwent single photon emission computed tomography (SPECT) scan at baseline and at regular intervals during the study. The primary outcome measure was the change from baseline in striatal [123I] -CIT uptake, a marker of dopamine neuron degeneration, at 46 months.

The percent loss in striatal -CIT uptake was significantly reduced in the pramipexole group compared to the levodopa group(~40%), suggesting slower disease progression in the pramipexole group compared to the levodopa group. However, direct pharmacologic effects of these medications, or compensatory mechanisms induced by them, cannot be excluded as possible alternative explanations for these results.

What is cabergoline?

Cabergoline (Cabaser®) is a long-acting ergot dopamine agonist with a high affinity for D2 receptors [70]. Its biological half-life is approximately sixty-five hours [71] and it is usually administered as a once a day dose. Cabergoline can be introduced at a dose of 0.05 mg and titrated to a usual maximum of 5 mg once daily. Side effects are similar to other agonists and include dizziness, somnolence, headache, nausea, and orthostatic hypotension [72].

In a six-month study comparing cabergoline to placebo as adjunctive therapy to levodopa for patients with motor fluctuations, cabergoline allowed an 18% reduction in levodopa dose compared with 3% in placebo-treated patients ($p < .001$) [73]. Motor function improved 16% in the cabergoline group compared with 6% in the control group ($p = .03$). ON time was significantly increased ($p = .02$) and associated with a corresponding decrease in OFF time and ON time with dyskinesia.

A double-blind, multi-center trial compared cabergoline and levodopa as initial therapy in 419 patients [74]. Patients were randomized to receive cabergoline or levodopa, underwent medication titration to an optimal dose up to week 24, and continued on this dose for up to five years. There was a significant delay in motor complications in the cabergoline group compared to the levodopa group (22.3% vs 33.7%). The relative risk of motor complications was >50% lower (0.46; $p < 0.001$) in the cabergoline group compared with the levodopa group. However, the levodopa-treated group had greater improvements in UPDRS motor scores.

There is concern that ergot dopamine agonists including cabergoline can cause fibrotic valvular heart disease [75]. However, a retrospective review of 234 PD cases from three centers in the UK found a low risk of fibrotic side effects with cabergoline, including cardiac valvulopathy [76]. Further prospective studies are needed to assess this risk.

What is Apomorphine?

Apomorphine (Apokyn®) is a non-ergot dopamine agonist that is approved for subcutaneous injection to treat acute intermittent hypomobility or OFF states. In the EU, it is also used as a continuous subcutaneous infusion (see chapter 9). It was suggested as a Parkinson's disease medication in the late 19th century, and clinical trials began in the 1950's [77,78]. Its early clinical use was limited due to untoward side effects, including nausea and hypotension. Apomorphine reemerged as a treatment for PD with the concomitant use of antiemetic medications that improved its tolerability.

Apomorphine has strong activity at both D1 and D2 receptors, and its half-life when administered parenterally is about 40 minutes. It is not currently available in an oral form due to extensive first-pass metabolism on oral administration [79]. Onset of action following subcutaneous injection is usually within ten to fifteen minutes and its effect lasts 90 to 120 minutes [80]. Because of its rapid onset of action, apomorphine subcutaneous injections are used as rescue therapy for refractory OFF periods. An antiemetic is usually administered for three days prior to its use in order to reduce nausea following injection, and the antiemetic is usually continued for at least six weeks

A prospective, double-blind, placebo-controlled study evaluated apomorphine in 29 advanced PD patients with two or more hours OFF time. Patients were randomly assigned patients to subcutaneous injections of apomorphine (2-10 mg, n = 20) or matched placebo (n = 9) during an inpatient and one-month outpatient phase [81]. During inpatient testing, apomorphine injection resulted in a reduction of mean UPDRS motor scores by 23.9 points (62%) compared to 0.1 point (1%) by placebo (P<.001). Ninety-five percent of outpatient injections resulted in reversal of the OFF state, compared to 23% of the placebo injections (P<.001). Patients taking apomorphine had a net reduction of two hours of OFF time per day. Adverse events include yawning, somnolence, dyskinesia, nausea and vomiting.

The optimal dose of apomorphine for subcutaneous injection must be determined individually for each patient. All patients should be pre-treated with an antiemetic prior to apomorphine initiation; in Europe, domperidone is used, while trimethobenzamide (Tigan®) 250 to 300 mg three times daily is used in the US. Patients are then brought to a doctor's office in the OFF state. Blood pressures are measured both in the lying and standing positions and then a test dose of apomorphine 2 mg (0.2 mL) is injected subcutaneously. Orthostatic blood pressures should be measured at 20, 40, and 60 minutes following the first test dose. If the patient has a good clinical response without untoward side effects, he or she may be sent home with instructions to subcutaneously inject 2 mg (0.2 ml) to reverse OFF periods [79]. If the patient does not respond to the 2 mg test dose, a test dose of 4 mg can be administered two hours after the initial test dose. A patient who tolerates 4 mg as a test dose should be sent home with a starting dose of 3 mg for OFF periods and the dose can then be increased by 1 mg increments every few days at home [79].

In clinical trials, most patients responded to 3 to 6 mg doses. The average frequency of dosing in the apomorphine development program was three times daily. There is limited experience with dosing frequencies higher than five times per day or total daily doses exceeding 20 mg (2 mL). Titration of apomorphine can alternatively be accomplished at home using 1 mg increments, to a maximum of 6 mg.
Many patients can discontinue the antiemetic six weeks after initiation of apomorphine injections.

Are there other dopamine agonists?

Lisuride is a hydrophilic semisynthetic ergot alkaloid dopamine agonist. It stimulates D2 and 5-HT (serotonin) receptors [82]. When given orally its half-life is one and a half to two hours. It is water-soluble and can also be administered subcutaneously or by continuous intravenous infusion to help ameliorate severe motor fluctuations [83,84].

What are the advantages of using dopamine agonists?

Rapidly fluctuating levels of levodopa-derived dopamine may sensitize dopamine receptors and lead to dyskinesia. Unlike levodopa, dopamine agonists directly stimulate post-synaptic dopamine receptors. They do not undergo oxidative metabolism and there is no evidence that they might accelerate the disease process.

Bromocriptine, pergolide, ropinirole, pramipexole, and cabergoline all have significantly longer half-lives than levodopa and do not expose receptors to rapidly fluctuating levels of stimulation. Several prospective studies have found that initial treatment with a dopamine agonist followed by the addition of levodopa when necessary is associated with a lower prevalence of dyskinesia [85,86].

The main limitation of dopamine agonist monotherapy is that symptoms are adequately controlled for a period of only one to five years. Rinne found that after three years of bromocriptine monotherapy only 28%, and after five years only 7%, of patients were still adequately maintained on monotherapy alone [87]. In the ropinirole five-year study, 54% of ropinirole-assigned patients remaining in the study at three years and 34% at five years were still on monotherapy [62]. After a few years, most patients require the addition of levodopa to sustain good benefit.

In moderate and advanced disease, dopamine agonists provide benefit for patients with motor fluctuations on levodopa therapy. When an agonist is added, OFF time is reduced, motor function is improved and levodopa doses may be reduced. Only rarely can a patient with fluctuations and dyskinesia on levodopa be adequately managed with dopamine agonists alone.

How do I switch from one dopamine agonist to another?

One can switch directly from one agonist to another by substituting potency equivalent doses. Alternatively, a patient can be tapered off one agonist before introducing another at a low dose and escalating upward. The mg potency ratio of the various agonists is: 10 mg bromocriptine = 1 mg of pergolide = 1 mg of pramipexole = 1 mg of cabergoline = 3 mg of ropinirole.

Can I abruptly stop dopaminergic medications?

Dopaminergic medications (levodopa preparations and dopamine agonists) should generally not be abruptly discontinued. Although many patients will tolerate abrupt withdrawal without difficulty, there is the possibility that a rare patient may experience neuroleptic malignant syndrome, a potentially fatal condition.

Is excessive daytime sleepiness related to dopamine agonist use?

Excessive daytime sleepiness (EDS) is a concern in PD patients as it may cause unintended episodes of sleep and lead to traffic accidents or other injuries. Patients should be questioned about sleepiness, and episodes of unintended sleep. In addition, the Epworth Sleepiness Scale can be a helpful screening tool.

Although EDS was initially attributed to pramipexole and ropinirole use[88], it is now clear that any dopaminergic medication can cause sleepiness, and other factors may also be involved. In a study of 638 highly functional PD patients without dementia in which 420 were active drivers, EDS was reported in 51% of patients and 51% of active drivers. There were no differences in sleepiness scores or the risk of falling asleep while driving with regard to the particular dopamine agonist used[89]. In a study of 303 PD patients, the factors most highly predictive of EDS were longer disease duration, more advanced disease, male gender and use of any dopamine agonist[54]. However, falling asleep while driving was best predicted by older age, use of levodopa, and use of any dopamine agonist[90].

It seems prudent that patients who doze off while driving or who fall asleep during activities such as working, eating or holding a conversation should not drive. If a particular medication can be identified that might be causing sleepiness consideration can be given to reducing or discontinuing it. It should also be recalled that PD patients do experience sleep disorders such as sleep apnea, and a polysomnogram can help identify these conditions.

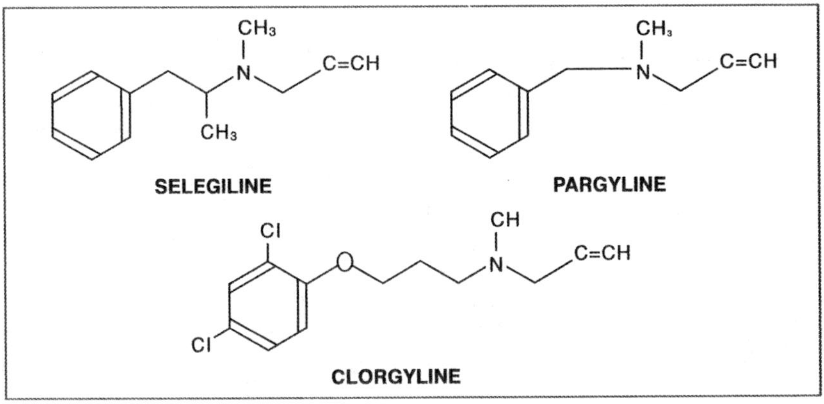

Figure 6.7. *Chemical structures of selegiline, a selective MAO-B inhibitor; pargyline, a non-selective MAO inhibitor; and clorgyline, a selective MAO-A inhibitor.*

Do dopamine agonists cause gambling?

A retrospective database review of PD patients over a one-year period found that nine patients had pathological gambling that was associated with high dose dopamine agonist use[91]. Eight of the patients were on pramipexole (mean dose

4.3 mg/day, range 2 to 8 mg/day), and one patient was on pergolide
(4.5 mg/day) at symptom onset. The incidence of pathological gambling was
1.5% in the pramipexole group and 0.3% in the pergolide group, while the
overall incidence was 0.05%. Another review identified 11 patients with
pathological gambling over a two-year period, and all were taking a dopamine
agonist [92]. Nine of the 11 patients were on pramipexole.

Pathologic gambling is one type of impulse control disorder. It appears likely that
other types of impulse control disorders can also be uncommonly related to
dopamine agonist use including excessive shopping (including online auction
sites) and inappropriate sexual behavior [93,94]. Patients should be warned about
these possible side effects when dopamine agonists are introduced and asked
about them during office visits. These behaviors usually resolve with reduction of
dose or discontinuation of the mediation.

What is selegiline?

Selegiline is a relatively selective, irreversible monoamine oxidase type B
(MAO-B) inhibitor (figure 6.7). In the brain, MAO-B is one of the enzymes
responsible for the clearance of dopamine. Selegiline boosts the symptomatic
effect of levodopa by slowing the breakdown of levodopa-derived dopamine in
the brain. In the research literature selegiline was known as deprenyl or
l-deprenyl. The standard dose is 5 mg with breakfast and lunch. Selegiline is
absorbed and crosses the blood-brain barrier without difficulty. The serum
half-lives of selegiline and its meatbolites are less than 24-hours [95]. However, the
clinical effect of selegiline may last months as resolution of its effect is
dependent on generation of new MAO-B in the brain.

How was selegiline created?

Selegiline was initially intended to be a "psychic energizer", created by
combining an amphetamine moiety with an antidepressant-like compound [96].
The development of MAO inhibitors began in the 1950s, when iproniazid,
an anti-tuberculosis agent, was found to improve depression. Early
antidepressants were difficult to use as MAO-A inhibitors were associated with
the risk of hypertensive crisis. Normally, MAO-A in the gut metabolizes ingested
amines such as tyramine and prevents their absorption. When MAO-A in the gut
is inhibited, ingested amines can be absorbed and may cause sympathomimetic
crises, sometimes called the "cheese effect". Manifestations of sympathomimetic
crisis include hypertension, vomiting, increased heart rate, and headache.

When gut MAO-A is inhibited, levodopa can cause sympathomimetic crisis as readily as tyramine. For this reason, levodopa preparations should not be given concurrently with MAO-A inhibitors. As a relatively selective MAO-B inhibitor, selegiline at recommended dosages can be safely administered with levodopa.

Selegiline is highly selective for inhibition of MAO-B in doses up to 10 mg per day [96]. Above 10 mg per day, it begins to lose its MAO-B selectivity and the risk of sympathomimetic crisis increases. Therefore, doses above 10 mg per day are generally not recommended.

What are the side effects of selegiline?

Selegiline is generally well tolerated. It is typically administered in the morning and at midday rather than in the evening to minimize the potential for insomnia. Some patients experience gastrointestinal side effects such as nausea [96]. When administered concurrently with levodopa, the most common side effect is an exacerbation of dopaminergic adverse effects. If a patient has peak-dose dyskinesias or hallucinations on levodopa, these may worsen with the addition of selegiline [97].

What medications should be avoided in patients who are taking selegiline?

A constellation of symptoms known as the serotonin syndrome may occur with the use of serotomimetic agents, taken alone or in combination with MAO inhibitors including selegiline. These agents include serotonin reuptake inhibitors, tricyclic and tetracyclic antidepressants, meperidine and other opiates, dextromethorphan, and tryptophan. The syndrome is characterized by various combinations of confusion, agitation, restlessness, rigidity, hyperreflexia, shivering, autonomic instability, myoclonus, coma, low grade fever, nausea, diarrhea, diaphoresis, flushing, and rarely rhabdomyolysis and death [98]. Patients taking selegiline should therefore avoid meperidine and other opiates.

The actual incidence of serious events when selegiline is used in combination with antidepressants is unknown. A chart review study did not identify any major side effects from combination therapy and serious interactions appear to be rare [99]. In clinical practice, antidepressants are commonly used at the same time as selegiline because many patients with Parkinson's disease require treatment for depression.

When should I use selegiline?

Selegiline is beneficial as an adjunct to levodopa for patients who are experiencing deterioration in the quality of their response. For patients with motor fluctuations, selegiline reduces OFF time and extends the short duration response of levodopa. In addition, selegiline provides modest symptomatic benefit as monotherapy in early PD and can delay the need for other symptomatic treatments[100].

Why was there interest in whether selegiline could slow disease progression?

The concept that selegiline might slow disease progression initially came from several observations. The ability of the neurotoxin MPTP to cause dopamine cell death and induce parkinsonian symptoms in animals and man is dependent on its oxidation to MPP+ by MAO-B. When selegiline is administered prior to MPTP, MPTP is not converted to MPP+ and parkinsonian symptoms are not elicited[101]. If there is an environmental neurotoxin similar to MPTP that causes Parkinson's disease in man, then selegiline might prevent its oxidation and protect against dopamine cell damage. Similarly, if free radical formation from the oxidative metabolism of dopamine by MAO-B contributes to disease progression, inhibition of MAO-B by selegiline may reduce free radical formation and slow dopamine cell degeneration.

What is the DATATOP study?

The Parkinson Study Group examined the ability of selegiline and tocopherol (vitamin E), alone or together, to slow the progression of Parkinson's disease. This was called the "Deprenyl and Tocopherol Antioxidative Therapy of Parkinsonism" study, or DATATOP. Eight hundred patients with early Parkinson's disease not yet requiring levodopa therapy were enrolled in the study. Subjects were randomized to one of four groups:

1) selegiline (10 mg/day) and tocopherol placebo,
2) tocopherol (2000 IU/day) and selegiline placebo,
3) selegiline and tocopherol,
4) selegiline placebo and tocopherol placebo.

The primary endpoint was the time required for the patient to develop sufficient disability to warrant the use of levodopa therapy. Results demonstrated that patients assigned to receive selegiline (alone or with tocopherol) experienced a significant delay in the need for levodopa therapy (hazard ratio = 0.50, p<0.001) (figure 6.8) [102].

Patients on selegiline placebo required levodopa at a projected median of 15 months from enrollment compared to 24 months for patients on selegiline. Tocopherol had no effect on the endpoint. This study demonstrates that the use of selegiline in early Parkinson's disease delays the need for levodopa therapy. However, the study also found that selegiline alone provided a small symptomatic benefit. It is not known if this delay in need for levodopa was due entirely or in part to this small symptomatic effect. A clear neuroprotective effect of selegiline has not been demonstrated in PD patients.

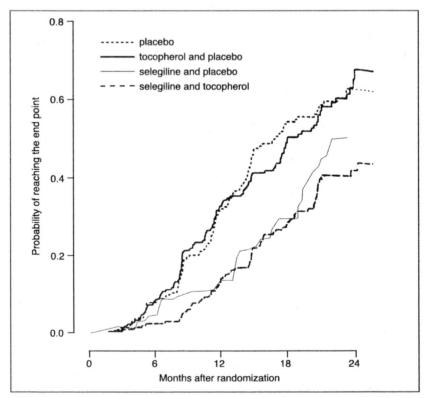

Figure 6.8. *DATATOP results. Kaplan-Meier estimate of the cumulative probability of reaching the end point, according to treatment group. The hazard ratio for patients assigned to selegiline compared to patients assigned to selegiline placebo with respect to the risk of reaching the endpoint per unit time is 0.50 (p<0.001; 95 percent confidence interval, 0.41 to 0.62).*

What is the role of selegiline in the treatment of Parkinson's disease?

Selegiline can be used in early Parkinson's disease to delay the need for levodopa and in advanced disease to decrease OFF time periods in patients with motor fluctuations. However, its symptomatic effects are generally modest.

What is Zydis selegiline?

Zydis selegiline is a wafer that dissolves in the mouth upon contact with saliva. It is absorbed in the mouth and bypasses hepatic first-pass metabolism. This route of absorption may allow higher plasma concentrations of selegiline compared to oral selegiline tablets.

In a double-blind, multi-center trial, 140 PD patients who were experiencing motor fluctuations on levcdopa were randomized to receive Zydis selegiline or placebo in a 2:1 ratio [103]. Treatment with Zydis selegiline 1.25 mg resulted in significant reductions in daily OFF time at four to six weeks (9.9%, p = 0.003) and at 10 to 12 weeks using the 2.5 mg dose (13.2%, p < 0.001). There was a reduction in the total number of OFF hours of 2.2 hours in the Zydis selegiline group compared with 0.6 hours in the placebo group. There was also an increase in the average number of dyskinesia-free ON hours (by 1.8 hours) in patients taking Zydis selegiline at week 12. Zydis selegiline was well-tolerated, safe and effective when used as adjunct therapy to levodopa in PD patients with motor fluctuations.

What is Rasagiline?

Rasagiline (N-propargyl-1(R)-aminoindan) is a second-generation, irreversible monoamine oxidase (MAO)-B inhibitor [104] that is administered once daily. It is five to 10 times more potent than selegiline, but unlike selegiline, is not metabolized to amphetamine-like derivatives. It provides a neuroprotective effect in a variety of cell culture and animal models. Rasagiline has been shown to effectively treat symptoms of Parkinson's disease when used as monotherapy in early disease and as an adjunct to levodopa in later disease [105-107].

One trial (the TEMPO study) evaluated the safety and efficacy of rasagiline in early PD patients in a multi-center, 26-week, double-blind, placebo-controlled trial [107]. Early PD patients numbering 404 who did not require dopaminergic therapy, were randomized to receive rasagiline 1 mg or 2 mg per day, or placebo. The primary outcome measure was the change in the total UPDRS score from baseline to study endpoint at 26 weeks. Both dosages of rasagiline significantly improved UPDRS

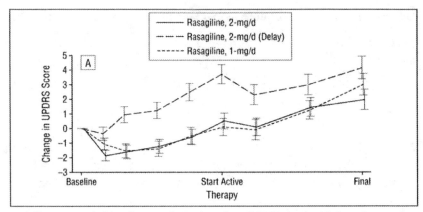

Rasigiline two month delayed-start study. Total unadjusted UPDRS score by visit for each treatment group for the 371 subjects included in the efficacy cohort. For the efficacy cohort, the last observation was carried forward for subjects with missing values for a given visit.
Arch Neurol, 2004, 61, 561-566. Copyright©(2004) America Media Association. All rights reserved.

scores compared to placebo. There were also significant improvements in motor and ADL subscales of the UPDRS in the active groups compared to placebo.

In the second phase of this study, patients who received placebo for the first six months were then treated with rasagiline 2 mg/day (delayed-start) while the other groups continued on rasagiline. Results demonstrated that at one year, patients treated with rasagiline from the beginning of the study were doing better than those who received placebo for the first six months. Patients treated with rasagiline 2 mg/day for the entire year exhibited a 2.29 unit smaller increase in total UPDRS score compared to patients who were treated with placebo for the first six months and rasagiline 2 mg/day for the second six months (p = .01). The delayed-start design was intended to distinguish a symptomatic effect of rasagiline from a neuroprotective effect. The results of the study suggest that rasagiline may slow disease progression but further investigation is required.

Another study (PRESTO) evaluated the safety, tolerability, and efficacy of the addition of rasagiline in levodopa-treated patients with motor fluctuations. This was a six month, multi-center, double-blind, placebo-controlled trial[106] in which 472 patients with at least 2.5 hours of OFF time per day were randomized to receive rasagiline 0.5 mg/day, rasagiline 1.0 mg/day, or placebo. The primary outcome variable was the change from baseline in total daily OFF time as assessed by patient home diaries. Results showed that patients treated with rasagiline 1.0 mg experienced a decrease in OFF time of 1.85 hours/day (29%), those treated with rasagiline 0.5 mg experienced a decrease in OFF time of 1.41 hours/day (23%), and patients treated with placebo experienced a decrease in

OFF time of 0.91 hours/day (15%). Thus, compared to placebo, rasagiline 0.5 mg/day reduced daily OFF time by 0.49 hours (p=.02) and rasagiline 1.0 mg/day reduced daily OFF time by 0.94 hours (p<.001).

In an 18-week, double-blind trial of patients with motor fluctuations on levodopa, the addition of rasagiline or entacapone was compared to placebo[108]. Patients were randomly assigned to rasagiline 1 mg once daily, entacapone 200 mg with every levodopa dose, or placebo. The primary outcome variable was the change in total daily OFF time. Rasagiline and entacapone both decreased mean daily OFF time, -1.18 hours for rasagiline (p=0.0001) and -1.2 hour for entacapone (p<0.0001) compared to -0.4 hours for placebo. In addition, rasagiline and entacapone both increased ON time without troublesome dyskinesia (0.85 hours vs placebo 0.03 hours; p=0.0005 for both). Both rasagiline and entacapone also improved activities of daily living UPDRS scores during OFF time and motor function scores during ON time.

What are anticholinergic medications?

Anticholinergic medications were the mainstay of anti-parkinsonian treatment until the latter part of this century. They are most effective for reducing tremor[109], and usually provide minimal benefit with regard to bradykinesia and rigidity. In addition, tremor may or may not improve with anticholinergic agents and a given patient may respond to one anticholinergic but not others. Their use is often limited by side effects and they are less well tolerated by older patients and those with dementia. Anticholinergics may cause confusion and hallucinations and most patients experience dry mouth or dry eyes[109]. Additional side effects may include urinary retention, ocular accommodation abnormalities, abnormal sweating, and tachycardia. Anticholinergics should be used with caution in patients with glaucoma. The most commonly used anticholinergic medications are trihexyphenidyl-HCl (Artane®) and benztropine mesylate (Cogentin®).

What is amantadine?

Amantadine (Symmetrel®), or 1-amino-adamantine is an antiviral medication, which was first found to improve symptoms in Parkinson's disease patients while being used to treat influenza in the 1960s. Subsequent trials confirmed that amantadine provides some benefit for the features of Parkinson's disease[110]. In addition, studies have demonstrated that amantadine can symptomatically reduce levodopa-induced peak-dose dyskinesias[111]. This effect has shown to be maintained for at least one year[112].

Although amantadine's exact mechanism of action is unknown, it appears to augment dopamine release, may inhibit dopamine reuptake and may stimulate dopamine receptors[113]. Amantadine is well absorbed and has a long half-life of approximately 24 hours. It is usually administered at a dose of 100 mg BID or TID. Because of its urinary excretion, it should be used with caution in patients with renal disease. Side effects include hallucinations, confusion, nightmares, ankle edema, dry mouth, and livedo reticularis, an erythematous rash of the lower extremities. Hyponatremia has also been described. Amantadine can readily exacerbate hallucinations and should be used cautiously in patients with dementia or prior hallucinations.

CHAPTER 7

MEDICAL MANAGEMENT OF PARKINSON'S DISEASE

Theresa A. Zesiewicz, Robert A. Hauser

What is the goal of medical management of Parkinson's disease?

The goal of medical management of Parkinson's disease is to adequately control signs and symptoms while minimizing side effects for as long as possible.

What are some general guidelines for the use of medications in Parkinson's disease?

It is recommended to make only one medication change at a time so that the positive and negative effects of that change are clear. Symptomatic medications should be initiated at a low dose and slowly escalated based on clinical response in order to minimize the incidence of early side effects. Signs and symptoms progress slowly and rapid medication changes are rarely required. Although knowledge and experience are useful guides, each patient must be assessed and treated as an individual.

Will medications eliminate the signs and symptoms of Parkinson's disease?

Except in very early disease, medications will not entirely eliminate signs and symptoms of Parkinson's disease. As the disease progresses, symptoms increase despite best medical management. Asymmetry often persists with worse signs apparent in the first-affected extremity.

How do I know if an increase in medication is warranted?

The presence of functional disability warrants a trial of increased medication therapy. Experience is the best guide to realistic expectations. Nonetheless, if symptom control is inadequate, an attempt to bring about improvement is warranted. If no improvement can be achieved before intolerable side effects emerge, the lowest medication dose that will maintain the current level of function is appropriate.

What is the general approach to the medical treatment of Parkinson's disease?

One attempts to provide adequate symptomatic control throughout the course of the disease. The younger and healthier the patient, the more aggressively we base our treatment on strategies designed to maximize function over the long-term. This may include the use of rasagiline as the initial medication, the use of a dopamine agonist prior to levodopa, and using entacapone when levodopa is first introduced. Rasagiline provides mild symptomatic benefit, is very well tolerated, should delay the need for levodopa, and may slow progression of disability. The use of a dopamine agonist prior to levodopa, and using entacapone when levodopa is first introduced provide more continuous dopamine receptor stimulation. Studies in PD patients have demonstrated that initiation of dopamine therapy with a dopamine agonist causes less motor fluctuations and dyskinesia than levodopa alone. The addition of entacapone at the time levodopa is inroduced has been demonstrated to cause less motor fluctuations and dyskinesia in the MPTP monkey model of PD. These approaches can be easily implemented without compromising symptomatic control.

In contrast, for older patients and those with cognitive impairment, focus is more on providing symptomatic benefit in the short to mid-term with the fewest side effects possible. For these patients we generally do not use dopamine agonists and depend more on levodopa.

When should one introduce symptomatic medication therapy for Parkinson's disease?

In general, it is recommended that symptomatic medications be initiated when the patient begins to experience functional disability. Patients with very early disease can be monitored clinically for the development of functional disability. Functional disability is present when symptoms of Parkinson's disease interfere with activities the patient either wants or needs to do. This should be assessed individually for each patient in the context of his/her lifestyle. A small loss of finger dexterity may threaten a keyboard operator's livelihood and warrant symptomatic therapy, whereas a retiree may have greater motor dysfunction without disability and may not require symptomatic therapy.

However, the TEMPO study that evaluated rasagiline in early PD, found that patients who started rasagiline early had less progression in UPDRS scores than subjects who took placebo for 6 months before starting rasagiline [1]. This suggests that with regard to rasagiline, consideration can be given to starting it before the patient experiences functional disability.

At the current time, there are no medications proven to slow the progression of the underlying disease. If such a "neuroprotective" medication were available, it would be started as soon as the diagnosis could be made.

What should I do when a patient develops functional disability?

Symptomatic therapy should be initiated when functional disability emerges. For many patients, especially those with younger-onset of symptoms, we begin dopaminergic therapy with a dopamine agonist. Dopamine agonists provide anti-parkinsonian benefit approximately equal to levodopa therapy for six months to a year and may adequately control symptoms for several years. Levodopa is added when agonist therapy alone no longer provides sufficient symptomatic benefit. By starting symptomatic therapy with a dopamine agonist one delays the need for levodopa and provides relatively smooth dopamine receptor stimulation.

Once levodopa therapy becomes necessary, one is able to use lower doses when it is administered concurrently with an agonist. There is good evidence to suggest that this approach is associated with a lower prevalence of motor fluctuations and dyskinesias [2-5].

One can then consider whether entacapone should be included as soon as levodopa therapy is introduced in order to provide relatively smoother dopamine stimulation. This can easily be accomplished through the use of levodopa/carbidopa/entacapone (Stalevo) as the levodopa formulation. This approach has been suggested by monkey studies and is currently being evaluated in the STRIDE-PD study that will determine whether Stalevo delays the onset of dyskinesia compared to standard levodopa/carbidopa, regardless of whether patients are already on a dopamine agonist.

For older-onset patients and those with dementia, more emphasis is placed on short to mid-term considerations and one may elect to use levodopa rather than a dopamine agonist as the first dopaminergic agent. We use the lowest levodopa dosage that will adequately control symptoms.

One may also elect to use levodopa as the first symptomatic agent for patients who are very immobile, bradykinetic, or rigid, and for those who require relatively rapid improvement. In appropriate cases, a dopamine agonist can then be introduced shortly thereafter when reasonable control of parkinsonian symptoms has been achieved.

How do you dose the dopamine agonists?

The agonists are best introduced at a low dose and slowly escalated. Reasonably high doses should be achieved before their utility is assessed. An opportunity for improvement may be lost if they are judged ineffective at low doses. The two most commonly used dopamine agonists are ropinirole and pramipexole. Ropinirole is commonly initiated at 0.25 mg TID for one week, 0.50 mg TID for the second week, 0.75 TID for the third week, 1.0 mg TID for the fourth week, 1.5 mg TID for the fifth week, 2 mg TID for the sixth week, 2.5 mg TID for the seventh week and 3.0 mg TID for the eighth week. Further dose adjustments are made at increments of 0.50 mg TID per week based on patient response up to a maximum recommended dose of 24 mg per day. Pramipexole is initiated at 0.125 mg TID for one week, 0.25 mg TID for the second week, and 0.50 mg TID the third week. Further dose adjustments are made in increments of 0.25 TID per week based on patient response up to a maximum recommended dose of 1.5 mg TID.

What should I do when dopamine agonist therapy no longer provides adequate symptomatic control?

Levodopa therapy is generally required when dopamine agonist therapy no longer provides adequate symptomatic control. The dopamine agonist can be continued and levodopa added. This may reduce the long-term incidence of motor complications [3-5].

What levodopa formulation should I use when levodopa therapy is first required?

Standard levodopa/carbidopa, levodopa/carbidopa CR, and levodopa/carbidopa/entacapone are equally effective in improving motor symptoms when levodopa is first required. Generic formulations of standard and CR levodopa/carbidopa are available and are less expensive than the brand formulations. Patients may find levodopa/carbidopa CR or levodopa/carbidopa/entacapone more convenient because fewer daily doses may be required. In addition, there is interest as to whether more continuous dopamine receptor stimulation as afforded by levodopa/carbidopa/entacapone can forestall the development of long-term complications including motor fluctuations and dyskinesia.

How do I dose levodopa?

It is helpful to introduce levodopa at a low dose and then escalate slowly to minimize the incidence of side effects. Standard carbidopa/levodopa can be introduced at a dose of one half of a 25/100 tablet per day and escalated to a target of either one half tablet QID or one tablet TID over one month. For carbidopa/levodopa CR, the initial target dose is 25/100 TID or 50/200 BID, usually starting with 100 mg levodopa per day and slowly increasing over a period of one to three weeks.

Levodopa/carbidopa/entacapone, when used as initial levodopa therapy, is usually initiated at a dose of one 50/12.5/200 mg tablet (50 mg levodopa) or one 100/25/200 mg tablet (100 mg levodopa) per day and increased by one tablet a day each week to a TID or QID schedule. Further escalations are undertaken based on clinical response.

What is the usual timeline for this long term strategy?

There is a lot of variability in the rate of progression of Parkinson's disease. Nonetheless, most patients will require symptomatic therapy within one to two years of symptom onset. Once functional disability emerges, a dopamine agonist will often control symptoms for another one to three years before levodopa is required.

How much levodopa is too much?

Most experts try to keep the levodopa dose below 500-600 mg per day for as long as possible. Despite this, patients should receive as much levodopa as is necessary to adequately control symptoms. If the patient has sufficient bradykinesia and rigidity to cause meaningful disability, the levodopa dose should be increased. There is no maximal levodopa dose, and some patients require relatively high doses (~1000 - 1500 mg levodopa or more) to achieve good benefit. At some point in a levodopa escalation, the patient will encounter an intolerable side effect and this defines "too much" levodopa for that patient. If the levodopa dose is escalated and no additional benefit occurs, the dose should be tapered down to the lowest dose that still provides the current level of benefit. Higher levodopa dosages that do not bring about additional benefit should be avoided.

What does it mean if there is no improvement when I add levodopa?

Almost all Parkinson's disease patients with sufficient bradykinesia and rigidity will experience improvement when levodopa therapy is introduced. There are several reasons why there may be no appreciable response. The dose may be too low, the diagnosis may be wrong, attention may be focused on the wrong symptoms, or symptoms may be so slight that improvement is hard to identify. Most Parkinson's disease patients experience noticeable improvement with 600 mg of levodopa per day or less. Much of this improvement is reduced bradykinesia and rigidity, and increased mobility and dexterity. If no improvement is noted, and symptoms remain prominent, the dose should be slowly escalated to tolerance or at least 1000 mg per day.

Improvement in bradykinesia and rigidity may be overlooked if too much attention is focused on tremor. Tremor may or may not respond to levodopa. If the patient has minimal difficulty with bradykinesia, rigidity, dexterity and mobility, improvement may be hard to detect. Patients with atypical parkinsonism usually do not benefit from levodopa therapy. In addition, patients who have been on levodopa for some time may be unaware of the benefit that it is providing. If there is a question as to whether levodopa is providing benefit, a temporary taper is often helpful to clarify whether it is helping.

How should I approach the treatment of tremor?

Tremor usually does not cause much functional disability in Parkinson's disease. We attempt to treat bradykinesia and rigidity with dopaminergic medications and then evaluate residual tremor. If a functionally disabling tremor persists or is the only manifestation of Parkinson's disease, an anticholinergic medication can be introduced. Tremor is variably responsive to levodopa, dopamine agonists and anticholinergic medications. In addition, tremor may respond to one anticholinergic but not another, so it is worth trying several (sequentially) if necessary. Patients with medically refractory, disabling tremor may benefit from a surgical procedure such as deep brain stimulation.

What if my patient can not tolerate levodopa?

The long term treatment of Parkinson's disease without levodopa is almost always less than satisfactory. When a patient has disabling parkinsonian symptoms it is very important to employ all conceivable strategies to try to achieve tolerability. Smaller doses than were previously used should be employed to reintroduce the medication. If necessary, a levodopa tablet can be crushed and one small chip per day used as the starting dose. If a patient has difficulty initiating levodopa therapy due to nausea, he should be instructed to take it immediately following a meal. If nausea persists, additional carbidopa or benserazide may be helpful.

Although 75 mg of carbidopa per day is usually sufficient to saturate peripheral decarboxylase, some patients will benefit from carbidopa in doses up to 200 mg per day. In some cases, a peripheral dopamine blocker such as domperidone will be required, and this is usually quite effective. For patients whose intolerability is due to orthostatic hypotension, fludrocortisone or midodrine may be beneficial.

Patients with a very clear diagnosis of Parkinson's disease and who cannot tolerate levodopa despite the measures described above may be considered for Deep Brain Stimulation surgery.

How can I treat motor fluctuations?

After several months to years of a stable response through the day, many patients on levodopa begin to experience motor fluctuations and notice that the benefit wears off after a few hours. It is usually relatively easy to reduce OFF time in a patient with motor fluctuations who is not experiencing peak-dose dyskinesia. Several different strategies, alone or in combination, can be used to provide more sustained dopaminergic therapy. Possible strategies include adding an MAO-B inhibitor, a dopamine agonist, or a COMT inhibitor, dosing levodopa more frequently, increasing the levodopa dose, or switching from standard to a long-acting preparation or levodopa/carbidopa/entacapone (figure 7.1). The patient should be alerted to the fact that increased dopaminergic therapy may cause or worsen peak-dose dyskinesia.

How do I manage patients with both motor fluctuations and dyskinesia?

Patients with both motor fluctuations and troublesome peak-dose dyskinesia can present a difficult management challenge. The goal of treatment for these patients is to provide as much good functional time through the day as possible. This is accomplished by maximizing ON time without troublesome dyskinesia. An attempt is made to reduce both OFF time and troublesome or disabling dyskinesia. An increase in dopaminergic therapy may increase dyskinesia and a decrease in dopaminergic therapy may increase OFF time. For many patients with severe fluctuations and dyskinesia, the best that can be done with medications is to balance OFF time and dyskinesia. The patient's relative preference for OFF time versus dyskinesia should be taken into account.

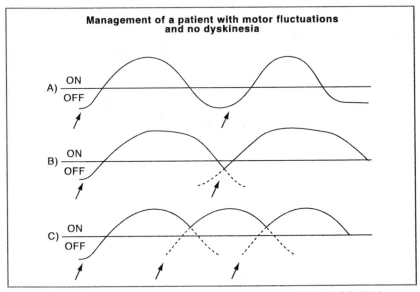

Figure 7.1. *Management of a patient with motor fluctuations and no dyskinesia (A). OFF time can be reduced by using a higher levodopa dose (B), switching to a long acting preparation or levodopa/carbidopa/entacapone (B), adding a dopamine agonist, or COMT or MAO-B inhibitor (B), or by shortening the interdose interval (C). Arrows indicate times of levodopa administration.*

Improvement is sought by attempting to provide as stable dopaminergic stimulation as possible within the therapeutic target zone. The addition of a dopamine agonist, or COMT or MAO-B inhibitor may be helpful. Dyskinesia may increase when these medications are added and downward titration of levodopa should then be undertaken. For patients on levodopa/carbidopa CR, it is often helpful to switch to a standard levodopa preparation to provide a more consistent and predictable dosing cycle (figure 7.2). It is then critical to titrate the dose based on clinical response. In general, it is desirable to administer smaller levodopa doses more frequently. A dose should be sought which is sufficient to turn the patient ON without causing too much dyskinesia (figure 7.3). The time to wearing-off then determines the appropriate interdose interval. Ideally, the next dose should be given to take effect when the previous dose begins to wear off. This can then be refined by the addition of a dopamine agonist, or COMT or MAO-B inhibitor, with possible additional titration of the levodopa dose, to further smooth the clinical response. In advanced disease, if a patient's response has become extremely erratic, he may have to take his next levodopa dose when he feels the previous dose wearing-off rather than adhering to a fixed dosing schedule.

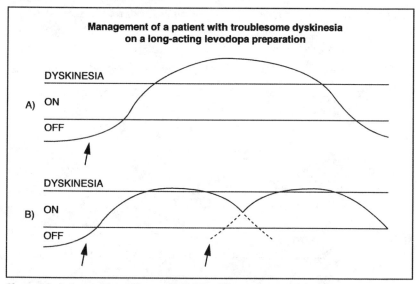

Figure 7.2. *Patients with troublesome dyskinesia while on a long-acting levodopa preparation (A) may benefit from a switch to standard levodopa/DDCI (B). This may allow for better titration and a more consistent dosing cycle. Arrows indicate times of levodopa administration.*

Another important treatment option for patients with fluctuations and dyskinesia is amantadine. Amantadine can both reduce OFF time and reduce dyskinesia [6,7]. Amantadine is initiated at a dose of 100 mg/day and can be escalated up to 400 mg daily. Its main disadvantage is that it relatively easily induces hallucinations and confusion and therefore should usually be avoided in patients with significant cognitive impairment or prior hallucinations.

What options are available for patients who have motor fluctuations and dyskinesias despite these treatments.

Apomorphine subcutaneous injections are available for patients with refractory OFF periods [8,9]. These injections are considered "rescue" therapy. They often provide symptomatic benefit in ten to fifteen minutes and last about an hour and a half. Side effects can include sleepiness and increased dyskinesia.

When medications are no longer effective in the management of motor fluctuations and dyskinesia, Deep Brain Stimulation should be considered.

Does diet play a role in motor fluctuations?

Levodopa competes with other large neutral amino acids for transport across the blood-brain barrier. Protein ingested in meals can slow levodopa flow into the brain. This usually has no impact on patients with relatively early disease, but can have a dramatic effect on patients with more advanced disease as

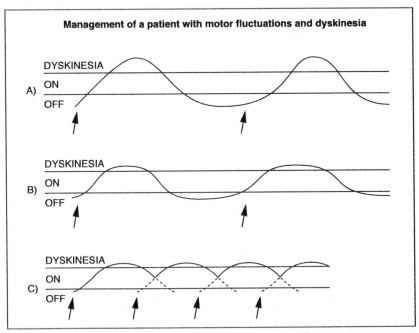

Figure 7.3. *The treatment of patients with motor fluctuations and peak-dose dyskinesia (A) generally involves providing less levodopa more frequently. The levodopa dose should be lowered until it brings on only mild dyskinesia (B). The time to wearing-off then determines the interdose interval (C). Arrows indicate times of levodopa administration.*

clinical status becomes critically dependent on continuous levodopa transport into the brain. Patients with severe fluctuations and those who find they turn off following a meal may benefit from a low protein or protein redistributed diet [10]. In addition, balanced carbohydrate-protein commercial food preparations are available. For patients with severe motor fluctuations, minimizing serum protein fluctuations may reduce the variability of levodopa transport and help provide a more stable clinical response.

How can I make levodopa take effect faster?

For patients with motor fluctuations, standard levodopa formulations commonly take 20-30 minutes or more before an effect is apparent. By chewing the tablet, the absorption rate is increased and clinical benefit occurs more rapidly. Another option is to dissolve the tablet in orange juice. This may be particularly useful for patients taking levodopa on an as needed basis when the previous dose has worn off and for patients who awaken immobile at night and need symptomatic benefit as quickly as possible.

What is liquid levodopa?

Patients with severe fluctuations and dyskinesia may gain some benefit when placed on a "liquid levodopa" regimen [11]. Patients are instructed to dissolve ten standard carbidopa/levodopa 25/100 tablets in one liter of water with one-half teaspoon of ascorbic acid. The result is a one mg per milliliter levodopa solution. The solution should be made fresh every day and hourly dosing is usually employed. An initial dosing schedule is calculated and further adjustments must be made to titrate to clinical response.

The first dose of the day is the same as had been taken in pill form. Initial hourly doses are calculated by dividing the patient's prior daily levodopa dose by the number of hourly doses he will be taking. When possible, the first daily dose is adjusted before the hourly doses. Adjustments are made in 5 mg increments every three to five days. Rather precise measurements are required for consistent dosing and many patients use a syringe to measure each dose. For successful initiation of liquid therapy it is critical to inform patients that the initial recommended schedule is only a rough guess as to dosing.

The ultimate benefit of a liquid regimen can only be assessed after optimal titration, which usually takes several weeks. Without this warning, patients are likely to abandon liquid therapy in the first few days when they experience increased OFF time or dyskinesia. Aggressive titration is vital. Most patients on liquid therapy use the levodopa solution through the day and take a levodopa/carbidopa CR or levodopa/carbidopa/entacapone tablet at bedtime to help them get through the night. Most patients find the liquid levodopa regimen rather cumbersome and abandon it after some time.

How do I treat wearing-off dystonia?

Wearing-off dystonia often responds to more sustained dopaminergic therapy. Substantial improvement is usually brought about by the addition of a dopamine agonist. Some patients benefit from a bedtime dose of a long acting levodopa preparation, switching to levodopa/carbidopa/entacapone, or the addition of a COMT inhibitor.

How do I treat diphasic dyskinesia?

Diphasic dyskinesia can be difficult to treat. In general, an attempt is made to increase and smooth dopaminergic stimulation. The goal is to avoid turning on and wearing-off as much as possible since these are the phases of the dosing cycle in which diphasic dyskinesia occurs. If medical therapy is not benefical, Deep Brain Stimulation can be considered.

What should I do if my patient is confused?

Dementia occurs in approximately 15-30% of Parkinson's disease patients[12]. It typically occurs late in the disease and progresses over time. Confusion can be exacerbated by medications. If confusion is present a review of all of the patient's medications is in order to identify those that are particularly associated with confusion. Any unnecessary medications should be discontinued. Any of the anti-parkinsonian medications can cause or exacerbate confusion. If confusion is evident, anti-parkinsonian medications should be reduced to see if improvement can be achieved.

One might first reduce and eliminate anticholinergics, and amantadine followed by reducing and eliminating the dopamine agonists. If necessary, the levodopa dose can be reduced. Patients with confusion may respond to cholinesterase inhibitors such as donepezil (Aricept®), rivastigmine (Exelon®), and galantamine (Razadyne®).

What should I do if my patient experiences hallucinations?

One must evaluate the impact of hallucinations. If the hallucinations are mild and non-bothersome, no change may be necessary. An attempt should be made to alleviate more severe hallucinations. Amantadine and anticholinergics, and if necessary, the dopamine agonists may be discontinued. If motor fluctuations are present, levodopa plus a COMT inhibitor may be the most useful combination.

If hallucinations are present on levodopa alone (with or without a COMT inhibitor) or if other medications cannot be reduced, an atypical neuroleptic can be added. Classical neuroleptics such as haloperidol reduce hallucinations but worsen motor symptoms. The preferred treatment is an atypical neuroleptic with minimal parkinsonian side effects. Quetiapine (Seroquel®) and Clozapine (Clozaril®) are useful to reduce hallucinations and have minimal parkinsonian side effects [13,14]. Some of the other atypical neuroleptics may have sufficient parkinsonian side effects to worse motor function in PD.

The most common side effect of clozapine is hypotension. The main serious side effect is the risk of neutropenia. Because of this risk, weekly monitoring of the patient's white blood cell count is required. The doses used to treat hallucinations in Parkinson's disease are much lower than those used to treat schizophrenia. Therapy can be initiated with one quarter of a 25 mg tablet at bedtime and slowly escalated every two to three days by one-quarter tablet until a beneficial dose is achieved. Most patients experience benefit at a dose of 25-75 mg per day.

Quetiapine is another atypical neuroleptic with minimal parkinsonian side effects [15]. It has become the treatment of choice for hallucinations in PD because it is not associated with agranulocytosis and blood monitoring is not required. Quetiapine is initiated at a dose of 25 mg at bedtime and escalated every week by 25 mg until a benefical dose is reached. The usual dosing range is 25-300 mg per day.

Clozapine and quetiapine are quite effective in reducing hallucinations but do not improve underlying dementia.

How can I treat Atypical Parkinsonism?

Anti-parkinsonian medications usually do not provide meaningful benefit for the clinical features of Atypical Parkinsonisms. Nonetheless, one can perform a levodopa trial, introducing it at a low dose and slowly escalating until intolerable side effects emerge. The goal is to achieve a levodopa dose of at least 1000 - 1500 mg to be satisfied that an adequate trial has been completed. If no benefit is realized, taper the dose downward to see if a loss of symptomatic benefit can be identified. When benefit occurs it is usually modest. Medication is discontinued if no benefit is identified. One of the reasons to perform a levodopa trial is to be sure not to miss a diagnosis of PD in a case with an unusual presentation and lose an opportunity for improvement. Much of the management of Atypical Parkinsonisms is supportive. Secondary symptoms such as depression and constipation should be identified and treated.

CHAPTER 8

NON-MOTOR SYMPTOMS OF PARKINSON'S DISEASE

Theresa A. Zesiewicz, Robert A. Hauser

What are the non-motor symptoms of Parkinson's disease?

Parkinson's disease (PD) is associated with non-motor as well as motor symptoms. Although the motor symptoms of Parkinson's disease (tremor, bradykinesia, rigidity, postural instability) are well-characterized, the non-motor symptoms are often described by patients as being more troublesome than the motor symptoms[1]. These symptoms are a major cause of PD morbidity, and are key factors in a patient's quality of life.

Unfortunately, non-motor symptoms are often under-recognized and under-treated, both in primary and secondary care settings[2-4]. One study found that depression, anxiety, fatigue, and sleep disturbances were not recognized in more than 50% of neurologic consultations for PD patients[5].

The non-motor symptoms of Parkinson's disease include:

SLEEPINESS AND SLEEP DISORDERS: excessive daytime sleepiness, unintended sleep episodes, insomnia, restless legs syndrome, sleep apnea, REM sleep behavior disorder, and vivid dreaming

FATIGUE: tiredness, lack of energy

AUTONOMIC DISTURBANCES: orthostatic hypotension, constipation, incomplete bowel emptying, fecal incontinence, dysphagia, choking, reflux, vomiting, nausea, heat intolerance, urinary symptoms (frequency, urgency, nocturia), sweating, hypersalivation, seborrhea, sexual dysfunction (hypersexuality, erectile dysfunction, impotence)

MOOD DISORDERS: depression, anxiety, apathy, anhedonia, obsessive behavior

COGNITIVE DISORDERS: Dementia, executive function abnormalities, psychosis

An international pilot study was performed to develop a comprehensive self-completed non-motor symptom questionnaire for Parkinson's disease [6,7].

Non-Movement Problems in Parkinson's Disease

Have you experienced any of the following in the last month?

1.	Dribbling saliva during the daytime	Yes	No
2.	Loss or change in your ability to taste or smell	Yes	No
3.	Difficulty swallowing food or drink or problems with choking	Yes	No
4.	Vomiting or feelings of sickness (nausea)	Yes	No
5.	Constipation (less than three bowel movements a week) or having to strain to pass a stool (feces)	Yes	No
6.	Bowel (fecal) incontinence	Yes	No
7.	Feeling that your bowel emptying is incomplete after having been to the toilet	Yes	No
8.	A sense of urgency to pass urine that makes you rush to the toilet	Yes	No
9.	Getting up regularly at night to pass urine	Yes	No
10.	Unexplained pains (not due to known conditions such as arthritis)	Yes	No
11.	Unexplained change in weight (not due to change in diet)	Yes	No
12.	Problems in remembering things that happened recently, or forgetting to do things	Yes	No
13.	Loss of interest in what is happening around you or in doing thing	Yes	No
14.	Seeing or hearing things that you know or are told are not there	Yes	No
15.	Difficulty concentrating or staying focused	Yes	No
16.	Feeling sad, "low" or "blue"	Yes	No

17.	Feeling anxious, frightened, or panicky	Yes	No
18.	Feeling less interested in sex or more interested in sex	Yes	No
19.	Finding it difficult to have sex when you try	Yes	No
20.	Feeling light-headed, dizzy, or weak when standing from sitting or lying	Yes	No
21.	Falling	Yes	No
22.	Finding it difficult to stay awake during activities such as working, driving, or eating	Yes	No
23.	Difficulty getting to sleep at night or staying asleep at night	Yes	No
24.	Intense, vivid dreams or frightening dreams	Yes	No
25.	Talking or moving about in your sleep as if you are 'acting out' a dream	Yes	No
26.	Unpleasant sensations in your legs at night or while resting, and a feeling that you need to move	Yes	No
27.	Swelling of your legs	Yes	No
28.	Excessive sweating	Yes	No
29.	Double vision	Yes	No
30.	Believing things are happening to you that other people say are not true	Yes	No

What casues excessive daytime sleepiness in PD?

Excessive daytime sleepiness (EDS) is sleepiness that occurs during the day and either causes an individual to take a nap or significantly interferes with activities of daily living. Up to 50% of PD patients experience EDS [8-10]. In PD, there are many causes and contributors to EDS, including the disease process itself, medications, and sleep disorders. Sleepiness in PD can be caused by degeneration of midbrain dopaminergic cell groups and their ascending pathways [11]. Sleepiness correlates with longer duration of PD ($p < 0.001$), more advanced PD ($p < 0.004$), and cognitive dysfunction [12].

A careful history may help pinpoint potentially treatable causes of EDS. Medications should be carefully reviewed to identify those that might be causing sleepiness. All of the dopaminergic medications can cause EDS, although dopamine agonists do so more frequently than levodopa [13,14]. In addition, anti-anxiety drugs, antidepressants, sedatives, anti-epileptics, and other medications can cause sleepiness. For patients who complain of sleepiness, the physician should review all medications being taken to determine those most likely causing sleepiness and to consider whether these medications can be reduce or discontinued.

Inadequate or poor quality overnight sleep also causes daytime sleepiness. In many cases this is caused by sleep disorders including insomnia, sleep apnea, REM behavior disorder, or restless legs syndrome. The physician should question the patient regarding how much sleep they get, how frequently they wake up, whether they feel refreshed in the morning, and whether their sleep appears peaceful to the bed partner or if there is snoring or excessive movement. If there is a suggestion of a sleep disorder, or if no cause for daytime sleepiness can be found, a sleep test (polysomnography) should be considered.

How common are sleep problems in PD?

Sleep difficulties occur in 50% to 98% of PD patients. In one study, almost 30% of PD patients admitted to using pharmaceutical sleeping aids, including hypnotics, sedatives, or antidepressants, to help them fall or stay asleep [15].

In a survey of PD patients, 88.5% complained of difficulty with sleep maintenance, and most awakened two to five times per night [16]. In moderately to severely disabled PD patients, the overall prevalence of insomnia was reported to be 80% [17].

How can a doctor tell if I have a sleep disorder?

If you are experiencing daytime sleepiness or disruptions of sleep, your doctor may order a polysomnogram (PSG), or sleep study. During this test, your sleep is monitored by EEG (electroencephalography), to determine how long you are asleep and what stages of sleep you are in. Your airflow and chest expansion are monitored to determine if you are breathing adequately while asleep. In addition, your muscles are monitored by EMG (electromyography) to determine if they are relaxed and quiet, as is the case during normal REM (rapid eye movement) sleep.

Sleepiness is also evaluated by determining your time to fall asleep during nap opportunities, a technique known as multiple sleep latency testing (MSLT). MSLT is usually conducted the day after the overnight sleep study.

What is restless legs syndrome?

Restless legs syndrome occurs in approximately 20% of PD patients[12]. Individuals with this disorder experience an urge to move the legs. This urge is often associated with uncomfortable sensations in the legs, and is worse at night and when lying in bed. The sensations are variably described as a creepy crawly sensation. The urge to move and the uncomfortable sensations are temporarily reduced or improved when the patient moves his legs. Many RLS patients find the sensations so uncomfortable that they can not sleep and end up walking around at night to relieve them.

The dopamine agonists, including ropinirole and pramipexole, are considered first line therapy for restless legs syndrome. Opioids and anticonvulsants have also been shown to be effective in the treatment of RLS, but should be used with some caution in PD patients due to side effects such as sleepiness and possible dependency with opioids.

What is obstructive sleep apnea?

Obstructive sleep apnea occurs in about 20% of PD patients[18]. In this disorder, airflow during sleep is intermittently absent or reduced despite respiratory effort. In the general population, patients with sleep apnea are commonly stocky or obese, snore during sleep, and do not feel refreshed in the morning. Whether these predictors apply to sleep apnea in PD is not yet known. The incidence of sleep apnea increases with increasing age. Treatment usually consists of wearing an airflow mask (continuous positive airway pressure, (CPAP) although many patients find it uncomfortable. In addition to disrupting sleep, untreated sleep apnea can cause high blood pressure and cardiovascular disease, weight gain, headache, and memory problems, so every effort should be made to adequately treat it.

What is REM behavior disorder?

REM behavior disorder is characterized by loss of atonia during REM (rapid eye movement) sleep when dreaming occurs. This leads to "acting out of dreams", including sleep talking, shouting, and intense, sometimes violent movements.

Patients may inadvertently injure their bed partners by punching or choking them[19], or by causing cuts, fractures, or bruises. RBD has been reported in 25% to 50% of PD patients and can precede the clinical onset of Parkinson's disease by several years[20,21]. The disorder usually presents in the sixth or seventh decade and may begin with verbal sleep activities including laughing, yelling, and talking during REM sleep. Animal models indicate that RBD may result from disruption of the dorsolateral pontine tegmental area (PTA), an area of the brain that can be affected very early in PD[22].

During normal REM sleep, voluntary muscles are quiet and relaxed. In RBD, polysomnography (PSG) demonstrates lack of this normal muscle atonia, and may reveal limb or body jerking and violent behavior[23]. Patients with RBD may benefit from the use of clonazepam (Klonopin) in dosages of 0.5-2 mg at bedtime.

What other sleep disturbances do Parkinson's disease patients experience, and how can these be treated?

Insomnia is common in PD. Patients describe both an inability to fall asleep and numerous nighttime awakenings. Some may have difficulty falling asleep due to depression or persistent tremor. Early awakenings may be caused by a reemergence of symptoms at night as daytime medications wear off. Reemergence of tremor may turn a light arousal into a complete awakening. Rigidity and akinesia can make it impossible to turn over in bed. Some patients develop a reversal of sleep wake patterns and may nap excessively during the day and remain awake at night.

For some patients, insomnia can be improved through the use of "sleep hygiene", or good sleep habits. This includes a consistent sleep schedule, reduction of daytime napping, regular physical exercise, and a healthy diet. Patients should avoid drugs such as alcohol, caffeine, tobacco, and other stimulant agents in the late afternoon and evening hours[24]. In addition, a careful review of all current medications should be undertaken to identify those that might be causing insomnia. These may include brochodilators, stimulants, antidepressants, and weight loss medications.

If nighttime awakenings are related to parkinsonian symptoms such as reduced movement, tremor, or dystonia, the use of extended release levodopa, levodopa/carbidopa/entacapone (Stalevo), or dopamine agonists can be helpful. If the patient awakens at night and cannot get back to sleep because he is OFF, a Parcopa tablet, or a standard levodopa tablet dissolved in orange juice or chewed and swallowed, may provide relief after some time. Another option is injection of subcutaneous apomorphine as this will generally provide benefit in approximately 10-15 minutes.

Depression and anxiety commonly occur in Parkinson's disease and can affect sleep. If a patient has depression or anxiety, the addition of an antidepressant or an anxiolytic can improve sleep quality. Some sleep problems may be related to nocturia. In these cases, the use of medications such as tolterodine (Detrol®) at bedtime can be helpful to reduce bladder spasms.

Finally, in some patients the use of hypnotics may be the only way to treat insomnia. In patients with difficulty falling asleep, short acting hypnotics such as zolpidem (Ambien®) or zaleplon (Sonata®) can be tried. In patients with difficulty staying asleep, longer acting agents such as eszopicione (Lunesta), temazepam (Restoril®), trazadone (Desyrel®), or mirtazapine (Remeron®) can be helpful, but hangover effects may cause drowsiness or falls in the morning.

What if no cause for sleepiness can be identified?

If no cause of EDS can be identified, or if a necessary medication is causing the EDS, a wake-promoting medication can be considered. Modafinil (Provigil) is a wake promoting agent that is effective to reduce EDS in narcolepsy. Preliminary information suggests that it is also effective to reduce sleepiness in PD [24,25]. In some patients the benefit is quite dramatic and in others there may be little or no response. A polysomnogram (PSG) may be considered prior to initiating modafinil to exclude sleep apnea and other sleep disorders.

What are "sleep attacks"?

A "sleep attack" describes "an event of overwhelming sleepiness that occurs without warning, or with a prodrome that is sufficiently short or overpowering to prevent the patient from taking appropriate protective measures". These may occur while a patient is eating, drinking, walking, working, or while driving a car [26].

The term "sleep attack" was originally used to describe sleep episodes in patients with narcolepsy but the term was largely dropped because such episodes are commonly preceded by a prodrome of sleepiness lasting seconds to minutes [27]. The term "sleep attack" re-emerged in 1999 when Frucht et al described sudden episodes of falling asleep that caused driving accidents in PD patients taking dopamine agonists[28]. Some experts have postulated that sleep episodes associated with dopaminergic medications are preceded by a prodrome of sleepiness for which individuals may be amnestic. It has been suggested that the term "unintended sleep episodes (USE)" more appropriately describes these events in that the word "attack" fails to recognize the background of sedation that may precede the onset of sleep[29].

Patients taking Parkinson's disease medications should be informed about the possibility of sleep attacks. They should be warned that driving could become hazardous if such an event were to occur. If they begin to become sleepy while driving, they should pull off the road quickly and call for assistance. Physicians should routinely ask patients whether they fall asleep at inappropriate times or places and patients should not drive if they are experiencing unintended sleep episodes. Dopaminergic antiparkinsonian medication may need to be decreased, or potentially discontinued to resolve such episodes.

I take Parkinson's disease medications, and have begun to experience vivid dreams at night. Why do these occur and is there any treatment for them?

Parkinson's disease patients may develop visual hallucinations at night. These patients frequently have preexisting sleep disorders, but medications used to treat Parkinson's disease can also cause nighttime hallucinations and vivid dreams. In one study, 48% of 126 Parkinson's disease patients had altered dream phenomena, and 26% had hallucinations or illusions[30]. 82 percent of patients with hallucinations or illusions also had some form of sleep disorder. The addition of atypical neuroleptics, including quetiapine or clozapine at bedtime may help with these problems.

Does fatigue occur in Parkinson's disease?

Fatigue is a disabling, poorly understood, and underdiagnosed symptom in Parkinson's disease[31]. It is more prevalent in Parkinson's disease patients than in age-matched controls[32], and is characterized by tiredness, weakness, and exhaustion[33]. There is no clear association between the presence or severity of fatigue and severity of motor symptoms, disease progression, or dosage or duration of medications used to treat Parkinson's disease[33]. Fatigue may occur in Parkinson's disease patients who are not depressed, and may precede the appearance of motor symptoms[31]. If depression is present it should be treated and associated fatigue may improve. Otherwise, little is know as to how to improve fatigue in PD. Modafinil and stimulant medications are sometimes tried but have not been well evaluated.

What are the autonomic disturbances associated with Parkinson's disease?

Autonomic dysfunction is an important cause of non-motor symptoms of Parkinson's disease. James Parkinson described some of these symptoms in his original essay. Autonomic abnormalities may include orthostatic hypotension (lightheadedness due to a drop in blood pressure upon standing), constipation, incomplete bowel emptying, fecal incontinence, dysphagia, choking, reflux, vomiting, nausea, heat intolerance, urinary symptoms (frequency, urgency, nocturia), sweating, hypersalivation, and seborrhea.

As many as 70 to 80% of Parkinson's disease patients experience some degree of autonomic dysfunction [34]. Many patients develop a loss of variation in heart rate interval (R-R) in response to postural changes [35]. This is indicative of parasympathetic system dysfunction. Lewy bodies have been found in the lateral hypothalamus in Parkinson's disease patients, an area important to regulation of the parasympathetic system [36]. Autonomic dysfunction may also be caused by abnormalities in the sympathetic ganglia. Treatment of autonomic dysfunction is symptomatic.

What is orthostatic hypotension, and how is it treated?

Orthostatic hypotension is defined as a drop of 30 mm Hg in systolic blood pressure or a drop of 20 mm Hg in mean blood pressure (diastolic plus one-third of the pulse pressure) when going from the supine to standing position. Patients usually complain of lightheadedness and if the orthostatic hypotension is severe, syncope can occur. Asymptomatic orthostatic hypotension does not require intervention but patients whose blood pressure is less than 80/50 mm Hg are usually symptomatic. Associated symptoms include syncope and presyncope but they may also be non-specific such as fatigue, unsteadiness, headache, neck tightness or cognitive slowing, especially in the elderly.

As a first step, unnecessary medications should be discontinued. The patient should drink eight or more glasses of fluid each day and liberally add salt (up to 150-250 mEq) to the diet. Pharmacologic treatment can be undertaken to increase intravascular volume with mineralocorticoids [37], or to increase vascular resistance through stimulation of alpha receptors [38,39]. The mineralocorticoid fludrocortisone (Florinef®) is introduced at a dose of 0.1 mg once or twice a day and can be increased to as high as 0.3 to 0.6 mg per day. Supine hypertension and dependent edema are common and not unexpected but care must be taken to avoid congestive heart failure.

Midodrine (ProAmatine®) is a peripherally acting alpha-1-agonist that produces vasoconstriction of both arterioles and venous capacitance vessels [40-42]. The initial recommended dosage is 2.5 mg BID or TID. The usual maintenance dose is 30 mg/day in divided doses, with a usual maximum of 40 mg/day. It is well absorbed orally and generally well tolerated. Side effects include scalp pruritus and tingling, pilomotor reactions, gastrointestinal complaints, headache, and dizziness [40]. Because it does not cross the blood-brain barrier, it is less likely to produce central nervous system side effects than ephedrine [42]. As a selective alpha-adrenergic agonist, it is relatively free of beta-adrenergic side effects and pulse rate usually does not increase [40]. Patients with supine hypertension on midodrine (>150/90), should be treated by elevating the head of the bed to a 30-degree incline. Several open label and double-blind studies have shown that midodrine effectively controls symptoms of orthostatic hypotension in most patients [38,43]. Refractory cases may respond to combination therapy with fludrocortisone [39]. Rarely, ergotamine tartrate (Cafergot®) is used in the treatment of orthostatic hypotension.

Do Parkinson's disease patients suffer from constipation?

Constipation occurs commonly in Parkinson's disease. In a study comparing colonic transit time between Parkinson's disease patients and age and sex-matched controls, Parkinson's disease patients had delayed colonic transit affecting all segments of the colon [44]. Additional studies have identified decreased basal anal sphincter pressures and a hyper-contractile external sphincter response [45-47]. Colonic abnormalities in Parkinson's disease may have both central and peripheral causes. Lewy bodies have been found in the myenteric plexus of the colon, suggesting that Parkinson's disease may affect the enteric nervous system. There is also a report of the presence of Lewy bodies in the neurons of the dorsal group of the nucleus intermediolateralis of the 3rd sacral segment of the spinal cord [48]. Anismus, or paradoxical contraction of the striated sphincter muscles during defecation, may be part of a focal dystonia. Administration of apomorphine has resulted in improved defecation, suggesting that these problems may be related to dopamine deficiency [49].

Basic treatment of constipation is aimed at increasing stool bulk by adding more fiber to the diet and by increasing daily liquid intake. Fiber intake can be increased by having the patient eat more fruits and raw vegetables, as well as products containing bran. Exercise may also be helpful in alleviating constipation. Anticholinergics that inhibit gastric motility and promote GI dryness should be discontinued. Despite these measures, many patients still complain of significant straining and hard stools. Stool softeners such as docusate sodium (Colace®) may be necessary.

Polyethylene glycol (Miralax®) is an osmotic agent that causes water to be retained with the stool. It softens the stool and increases the frequency of bowel movements. The usual dose is 17 grams (one heaping tablespoon) of powder per day in eight ounces of water, soda, or juice. One study found that Tegaserod (Zelnorm®) provided modest improvement in constipation[50], while another study reported that mosapride citrate, a novel selective 5-HT4 receptor agonist, improved bowel frequency in parkinsonian patients and augmented lower gastrointestinal tract motility[51].

For patients with refractory constipation, lactulose preparations may be required. When possible, the long-term use of pharmacologic agents in treating constipation should be avoided. The simplest measures are best-tolerated long-term.

How can I treat dysphagia?

Dysphagia is also common in Parkinson's disease and patients often describe a "choking" sensation along with difficulty swallowing foods. Parkinson's disease can cause esophageal dysfunction and abnormalities in the oropharyngeal phase of swallowing. In one study of swallowing disorders in asymptomatic elderly patients with Parkinson's disease, videofluoroscopy was performed to evaluate facial, tongue, and palatopharyngeal musculature[52]. Although these patients denied any dysphagic symptoms, all patients had at least one abnormality of the swallowing mechanism. Oropharyngeal transit time was increased and patients needed more swallows to remove the bolus from the pharynx.

Lewy bodies have been found in the myenteric plexus in the esophagus in dysphagic Parkinson's disease patients[53], again suggesting that the enteric nervous system is affected. Radionucleotide motility studies have revealed slow transit time and demonstrated that dysphagia may improve with antiparkinson medication[54]. Dysphagia may increase the risk of aspiration, although one study failed to demonstrate increased rates of pulmonary infection in Parkinson's disease patients with dysphagia[55].

Parkinson's disease patients with dysphagia should eliminate hard foods from the diet and pay careful attention to swallowing. Increased dopaminergic therapy with levodopa may improve swallowing [56]. For patients with clinically significant dysphagia it is worthwhile to slowly increase the levodopa dose to tolerance to evaluate whether any improvement in dysphagia can be achieved.

How should I approach urinary incontinence in Parkinson's disease?

Patients complaining of urinary symptoms should have a urologic evaluation including cystometric studies to exclude other causes of urinary symptoms, including prostate abnormalities. Decreased levels of dopamine can cause detrusor hyperreflexia in Parkinson's disease patients, resulting in urinary frequency, urgency, and most commonly nocturia. A high incidence of instability of the detrusor muscles has been reported in incontinent Parkinson's disease patients [57].

A simple reduction in fluids after dinner may help to reduce nocturia [57]. Otherwise, use of an anticholinergic medication such as tolterodine tartrate (Detrol®, Detrol LA®), oxybutinin chloride (Ditropan®, Ditropan XL®) or propantheline bromide (Pro-Banthine®, Propanthel®) may be helpful. Tolterodine long acting is given in dosages of 4 mg once a day and the immediate release is given in dosages of 2 mg twice a day, oxybutinin is given in dosages of 5 to 10 mg at bedtime, and propantheline is administered in dosages of 15 to 30 mg at bedtime. Patients should be monitored for cognitive side effects. Of these medications, tolterodine is least likely to cause cognitive side effects.

If detrusor hypoactivity is present, a reduction in anticholinergic medications may be warranted. The use of desmopressin nasal spray to treat nocturia in Parkinson's disease has been explored. It may be considered for patients with significant adverse impact due to nocturia refractory to other measures [58], as electrolyte imbalance is a possible side effect.

How can I treat drooling?

It is estimated that 70% of Parkinson's disease patients eventually experience drooling [59]. Siallorhea in Parkinson's disease is caused by saliva pooling in the mouth secondary to swallowing difficulties, rather than from increased production of saliva [60]. Besides being bothersome to the patient, siallorhea can lead to more serious problems including chemical dermatitis or aspiration.

For some patients, increased dopaminergic therapy is useful to improve swallowing and reduce drooling. Anticholinergic medications can reduce saliva production, but may cause side effects including dry mouth, constipation, and cognitive changes. The peripheral anticholinergic glycopyrrolate (Robinul®) may be particularly useful to avoid cognitive side effects. More recently, injections of botulinum toxin into salivary glands have been described as an effective treatment for drooling. For the most difficult cases, salivary duct sclerosis may be considered. An open-label pilot study found that sublingual atropine drops subjectively and objectively reduced saliva production [61]. However, cognitive side effects can occur. Six PD patients and one PSP patient were tested; one patient experienced delirium, and two had worsening of hallucinations.

How should I treat seborrhea?

It is not uncommon to find excessive oiliness, chafing and redness of the skin, particularly of the forehead and scalp, in Parkinson's disease patients. Dandruff shampoos containing salicylic acid and coal tars can help with itching and flaking. Hydrocortisone cream 1% can be obtained over-the-counter and can be helpful if applied to the scalp or affected skin areas once or twice daily. Ketoconazole (Nizoral®) is available as a prescription cream or shampoo and can be helpful in some cases. The cream is applied to the skin twice daily for up to four weeks and the shampoo is used twice weekly for four weeks. If clinically warranted, the use of topical steroids may be beneficial. If there is an inadequate response, referral to a dermatologist for further evaluation and treatment is appropriate. There is some evidence that optimum dopaminergic management may reduce seborrhea [62].

How can I approach sexual dysfunction in Parkinson's disease?

Sexual dysfunction can occur for a variety of reasons including lack of mobility, loss of interest, or difficulty achieving and maintaining an erection. Nonetheless, the exact pathophysiology of sexual dysfunction is largely unknown. Loss of sexual interest is commonly reported in Parkinson's disease patients, and both men and women are affected. However, one study suggested that loss of sexual interest, although common, is no greater than that which occurs in other non-neurologic chronic diseases [63]. Depression and use of medications such as propranolol and other antihypertensives can contribute to sexual dysfunction [64,65]. After discontinuation of potentially offending medications and treatment of depression, a patient complaining of sexual dysfunction should be evaluated by a urologist to exclude other causes and direct further management.

Sildenafil citrate (Viagra®) is a phosphodiesterase type V inhibitor used to treat erectile dysfunction. In one open-label study of sildenafil citrate use in men with PD and erectile dysfunction, there were significant improvements in total Sexual Health Inventory Scores, overall sexual satisfaction, satisfaction with sexual desire, ability to achieve erection, ability to maintain an erection, and ability to reach orgasm [66]. No changes were noted in motor function with sildenafil citrate use.

How common is depression in Parkinson's disease patients?

Depression is the most commonly encountered "psychiatric" symptom in Parkinson's disease, affecting as many as 40 to 50% of patients. Parkinson's disease patients experience major depression more frequently than the normal elderly, and are significantly more depressed than nonparkinsonian control patients with comparable disability [67,68]. Depressed Parkinson's disease patients may meet clinical criteria for either major depression or dysthymic disorder [68,69] and often have concurrent symptoms of panic and anxiety [70]. In Parkinson's disease, depression is more commonly associated with dysphoria and sadness, rather than self-blame or guilt [72]. Most studies have not found an association between depression and severity or duration of illness, age, or gender [71]. It can occur at any time during the course of the disease and may emerge prior to motor symptoms. Depression may sometimes be difficult to diagnose in a Parkinson's disease patient because symptoms of depression and Parkinson's disease may overlap (sleep disturbance, weight loss, motor slowing, loss of motivation, and decreased libido).

Scales such as the Beck's Depression Inventory [73] and the Hamilton Depression Rating Scale (HDRS) [74] are used to assess depression in Parkinson's disease patients.

It is unclear whether the etiology of depression in Parkinson's disease is endogenous, reactive, or both. There is evidence that depression in Parkinson's disease is related to serotonergic abnormalities [75]. Nonetheless, it appears likely that both neurochemical changes and psychosocial issues may contribute to the development of depression in Parkinson's disease.

Antidepressants have been found to improve depression in Parkinson's disease patients in a limited number of studies [76-78]. Tricyclic antidepressants, such as amitryptiline (Elavil®), serotonin reuptake inhibitors, and atypical antidepressants have all been found to improve depression in Parkinson's disease. However, several case reports have noted worsening of parkinsonian symptoms after treatment with the serotonin reuptake inhibitors fluoxetine (Prozac®) and paroxetine (Paxil®) [79,80]. An open label study of sertraline (Zoloft®) found that it reduced depression in stable Parkinson's disease patients without worsening motor symptoms [81].

Patients who experience depressed mood only when levodopa wears off may benefit from strategies that smooth dopamine replacement therapy and may not require antidepressants.

What is the serotonin syndrome?

Selective serotonin reuptake inhibitors (SSRI's) are commonly used to treat depression in Parkinson's disease. However, SSRI's, either alone or in combination with monoamine oxidase inhibitors such as selegiline or rasagiline, can cause the "serotonin syndrome", characterized by mental status changes, tremor, diaphoresis, and incoordination. Deaths have occurred due to rhabdomyolysis, disseminated intravascular coagulation, respiratory distress syndrome, and cardiovascular collapse [82-84]. Treatment of the serotonin syndrome involves discontinuation of the inciting drug and supportive measures, with resolution of symptoms usually occurring in hours to weeks [85].

The occurrence of serotonin syndrome in Parkinson's disease patients receiving both selegiline and SSRI's is rare. A retrospective chart review evaluating the concomitant use of fluoxetine and selegiline failed to uncover any serious side effects or additional adverse events which had not already been reported with each medication alone [86]. A survey of physicians in the Parkinson Study Group (PSG) indicates that the combined use of selegiline and antidepressants rarely results in serious adverse events [87]. In addition, serotonin syndrome was not observed in clinical trials of rasagiline in which concomitant antidepressants were permitted in low dosages.

Does anxiety occur in Parkinson's disease?

Anxiety may affect 40% to 50% of Parkinson's disease patients, and may occur in association with depression. PD patients may also experience panic attacks [88]. Anxiety may also occur during OFF periods, when Parkinson's disease medications are not working [89].

Does dementia occur in Parkinson's disease patients?

Dementia is defined as a loss of intellectual abilities of sufficient severity to interfere with social or occupational functioning. Dementia is fairly common in Parkinson's disease. Reported prevalence rates range from 10% to 80%, but actual rates are probably closer to 40% [90,91]. Dementia usually emerges late in the course of PD, often after eight to ten years. One study found that PD patients who developed dementia were older at disease onset and had a longer duration of disease [90].

Dementia in Parkinson's disease can manifest as difficulty with memory, attention, problem solving, and personality and behavioral changes. Patients may also have impaired visuospatial function, and decreased verbal fluency [92]. There may be increased processing time with longer response latencies. Short-term memory may be specifically affected in patients with Parkinson's disease, while immediate recall and long-term memory remain fairly intact [93]. PD patients who suffer from dementia are at increased risk for nursing home placement [94].

The presence of dementia in PD is highly correlated with the presence of Lewy bodies staining for alpha-synuclein in the cortex [95]. This suggests that the same disease process that is causing loss of nigrostriatal dopamine neurons is occurring in the cortex of patients with dementia. Why this occurs in some PD cases but not others is not known. Alzheimer's disease pathology is found in only a small minority of PD patients with dementia.

One double-blind study evaluated the effect of donepezil (Aricept®) in 22 Parkinson's disease patients with dementia [96], and found that patients treated with donepezil 5 to 10 mg/day had improvements in the Mini Mental Status Exam (MMSE) and Clinical Global Impression (CGI) scale compared to patients treated with placebo. However, scores on the Assessment Scale-Cognitive Subscale (ADAScog) were not significantly different between the groups. There is some evidence that rivastigmine (Exelon) may improve cognitive dysfunction in Parkinson's disease [97].

Can Parkinson's disease patients develop psychosis?

Psychosis may occur in up to one-third of Parkinson's disease patients[98]. Symptoms include visual, auditory, or tactile hallucinations, paranoid delusions, and frank psychosis. Psychosis usually occurs later in the disease, and may be worsened by Parkinson's disease medications, including amantadine, dopamine agonists, anticholinergics, levodopa, MAO-B inhibitors, and COMT-inhibitors [99]. Risk factors for the development of psychosis include the presence of dementia, protracted sleep disorders, and a history of depression [100]. Daytime hallucinations often take the form of seeing people or animals. The presence of psychosis in Parkinson's disease may warrant a reduction in medication dose, or even the elimination of some medications. If symptoms persist, or drugs cannot be reduced or weaned due to motor symptoms, a trial of atypical antipsychotics may be necessary. Quetiapine (Seroquel®), and clozapine (Clozaril®) have minimal parkinsonian side effects and are quite useful to treat hallucinations [99]. Clozapine requires blood count monitoring.

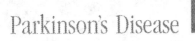

CHAPTER 9

THE EUROPEAN PERSPECTIVE ON THE TREATMENT OF PARKINSON`S DISEASE

Elisabeth Wolf, Werner Poewe

Parkinson's disease (PD) is a universal illness although prevalence rates in some parts of the world, including China and parts of Africa, seem to be lower than those in North America. In Europe, available data suggest a very similar prevalence and incidence to North America and approaches to diagnosis and management of PD are also generally very similar in Europe and North America. Nevertheless, subtle differences exist in management approaches, primarily related to the use of drugs that are licensed in the European market only but also regarding preferential use of some interventions over others in Europe as opposed to North America.

Although levodopa treatment continues to be the "gold standard" of symptomatic therapy both in North America and Europe, there are some differences in the types of levodopa preparations used. In addition, there are dopamine agonists on the European market that are not currently available in the United States. For the dopamine agonist apomorphine, which is available in both markets, modes of administration differ.

How is levodopa used in Europe?

As in North America also in Europe a number of levodopa formulations based on the combination with the peripheral dopadecarboxylase inhibitor carbidopa are available in regulary clinical use. Most recently levodopa/carbidopa/entacapone in one formulation has been added to this list. Differential from the US a second levodopa preparation based on a combination with the peripheral dopadecarboxylase inhibitor benserazide is also widely used. The corresponding preparation (Madopar) was originally marketed in Europe in the 1970's. It is available in various generic forms with dose sizes of 50/12.5 mg, 100/25 mg levodopa/benserazide. Like levodopa/carbidopa, the most common initial target dose is 100/25 3 times daily starting with 50/12.5 single doses per day and increasing by 50/12.5 at intervals between 2 and 7 days until the target dose is reached.

As with initiation of dopamine agonist therapy (see below), nausea complicating initial titration is treated with the peripheral dopamine receptor blocking agent domperidone (Motilium®), which is not available in the US. Domperidone is a benzamide derivate which, at usual recommended doses, does not cross the blood-brain barrier. Its antiemetic effect is based on blockade of dopamine-receptors in the chemoemetic trigger zone of the area postrema, which does not have a blood-brain barrier. In addition, it increases rhythmic contraction of the stomach, which shortens gastric emptying time. Several studies have demonstrated the beneficial effects of domperidone on levodopa or dopamine-agonist induced nausea and one study has shown reduced gastric emptying time[1]. Usually, daily doses range from 20-60 mg, given in three divided doses 15 to 30 minutes prior to intake of levodopa or apomorphine.

There are several alternative formulations of levodopa/benserazide available and used in Europe:

- A controlled release preparation of levodopa/benserazide (Madopar CR®) is available in a single dose strength of 100/25 mg capsules. The controlled release activity is based on a "floating capsule" principle where active drug is slowly released from a gelatinous matrix as the capsule remains floating on the gastric fluid for up to 12 hours. Bioavailability over standard levodopa/benserazide is reduced to about 60 % to 70 % and plasma level peaks as well as onset of clinical effect are delayed[2]. The primary use of levodopa/benserazide controlled release capsules is as a bedtime or nocturnal dose to counteract nocturnal immobility or early morning akinesia[3].

- A dual-release preparation of levodopa/benserazide is currently marketed in Switzerland. This formulation was created in an attempt to combine the short-latency onset of effect of standard levodopa/benserazide with the extended release duration in one pill. Descombes et al[4] recently reported results of a randomized, double-blind single dose study comparing 200 mg of levodopa plus 50 mg of benserazide given either as a slow-release or novel dual-release preparation consisting of a three layer tablet combining immediate and slow-release properties. Sixteen patients with PD and motor fluctuations were studied regarding time to switch "on", duration of "on", degree of UPDRS improvement and dyskinesia severity. In addition, pharmacokinetic parameters were compared.

The dual-release formulation resulted in significantly shorter times to switch "on" (43 vs. 81 minutes, p = 0.0009) compared to the slow-release formulation and there was a trend to longer "on" duration (114 vs. 80 minutes, p = 0.07). UPDRS improvement and dyskinesia scores were similar following administration of either preparation. C_{max} and AUC were significantly greater with the dual-release tablet and t_{max} was significantly shorter. There were no differences in tolerability. This preparation is the most commonly employed first line strategy to treat patients with early wearing-off in Switzerland.

- A third alternative delivery formulation of levodopa/benserazide is a dispersible tablet available in a 100/25 mg dose form that allows faster gastrointestinal absorption of levodopa, shorter times to peak plasma concentrations, and faster onset of clinical effect. Contin et al[5] studied pharmacokinetics and time to onset of the clinical response as assessed by a finger tapping test in a randomized cross-over single dose study comparing standard versus dispersible levodopa/benserazide in eight patients. Time to peak plasma levels (t_{max}) was significantly shorter after ingestion of the dispersible versus the standard formulation (median of 37 min. vs. 82 min., p < 0.02).

Clinical response parameters, however, were not different, except for a trend of shorter latencies to onset of motor response, which failed to reach statistical significance. Such preparations are commonly used to counteract delayed-ON-phenomena, either as the first morning dose or during the day. They are also sometimes prescribed on an "as required" basis as a rescue medication in patients with unpredictable motor response fluctuations.

Can levodopa be given as truly continuous delivery?

Constant delivery of levodopa has been demonstrated to stabilize motor performance in advanced patients. This was initially shown in pilot-studies using intravenous (i.v.) infusion of levodopa in patients with advanced PD and refractory response fluctuations[6, 7]. Due to the poor water solubility of levodopa and the low pH of solutions used for infusion, this requires a central line and is thus not practically feasible.

Duodenal absorption of levodopa is rapid and almost complete, and duodenal infusion of levodopa produces pharmacokinetic profiles similar to i.v infusions[8]. Kurth et al[9] compared duodenal infusions of levodopa/carbidopa versus standard oral dosing by exposing 10 patients with motor fluctuations to either regimen over two days in random sequence. Plasma levels were markedly more constant with duodenal infusions and functional "on" hours were also significantly increased during infusion days. Several open-label studies in small numbers of patients, including one report with a 10-year follow-up, suggest sustained clinical benefit from duodenal levodopa infusions in PD patients with motor fluctuations and some trials also report improvements in pre-existing dyskinesias [10].

In a recent report, Nyholm et al [11] compared oral levodopa treatment to levodopa infusions administered via nasoduodenal tubes in 24 PD patients in a randomized crossover study. They found significantly increased "on" time and corresponding decreases in "off" time with infusion therapy compared to conventional oral treatment without increasing dyskinesias. A new galenic formulation of levodopa, developed for intraduodenal administration, was recently introduced into the European market. The formulation is a stable suspension of levodopa (20 mg/ml) and carbidopa (5 mg/ml) in a methylcellulose gel (DUODOPA®). This levodopa gel is available in prefilled systems containing 100 ml (2000 mg).

Treatment requires percutaneous endoscopic gastrostomy (PEG) with a duodenal tube connected to a portable infusion pump designed for levodopa infusions (CADD-Legacy Duodopa pump®). The levodopa infusion is usually given during daytime, starting with a morning bolus dose. One study of 24-hour enteral levodopa infusion reported a shift of the dose-response curve to the right suggesting a trend to tolerance as a result of the round-the-clock infusions, whereas daytime infusions may have the opposite effect, showing increased sensitivity to levodopa with time [12]. Daily doses range from 20 to 200 mg/hour. Side effects of levodopa infusions seem to be equivalent to side effects of oral therapy. Also, local complications from the gastrostomy (local granulation, infection, segregation) have occasionally been reported. Dislocations of the duodenal tube had occurred frequently, leading to the development of a new self-propelling tube [13].

Which dopamine agonists are used in Europe that are not available in the US?

While the most commonly prescribed new non-ergot dopamine agonists ropinirole and pramipexole are first line agents both in North America and Europe, some dopamine agonists are currently only available in Europe and not in the US.

CABERGOLINE is an orally administered synthetic tetracyclic ergoline derivative that acts in vitro and in vivo as a selective D2 receptor agonist with no substantial affinity for D1 receptors. As with other ergotamine derivatives, it has also some affinity for non-dopamine receptors (noradrenergic and serotonergic).

A unique characteristic of cabergoline is its long elimination half-life of approximately 65 hours. Cabergoline is highly effective in suppressing prolactin levels (a dopaminergic effect) with a duration of action up to 21 days after a single 1 mg oral dose. This pharmacokinetic profile allows it to be administered as a once-daily treatment. The cabergoline t_{max} is observed at 2.5 hours, and it is metabolized into several metabolites excreted mainly in the feces. All clinical studies published on cabergoline used a once-daily dosing regime, however in clinical practice, an additional evening dose is sometimes administered, especially in PD patients with nocturnal disability. The recommended dosage for cabergoline is 2-6mg daily, with a starting dosage of 1 mg and increasing by 0.5-1 mg in seven-day intervals.

One randomized, double blind study published by Rinne et al[14] showed a similar effect on motor symptoms of cabergoline compared to levodopa at the one-year analysis. After three to five years, 35% of cabergoline treated patients still did not require levodopa therapy[15]. Two trials reported beneficial effects of cabergoline in advanced PD patients with fluctuations on levodopa[16,17]. Both studies, one comparing cabergoline to placebo and one comparing cabergoline to bromocriptine, showed a decrease of daily off time with cabergoline therapy.

Cabergoline induced side effects are consistent with adverse reactions reported with other dopamine agonists. There are a few reports of cabergoline induced pleural fibrosis and also some recent reports of cabergoline induced fibrotic valvulopathy[18,19]. In addition, a recent series found increased incidence of valvular regurgitation in PD patients treated with cabergoline compared to normal controls[20]. Therefore, echocardiographic safety monitoring seems advisable.

DIHYDROERGOCRYPTINE (α-DHEC) is a dihydro-derivative of ergocryptine acting as a D_2 agonist and a partial D_1 agonist. Therefore, DHEC has a pharmacodynamic profile comparable to that of bromocriptine. It has a half-life of about 16 hours. Like all ergotamine derivatives, DHEC has effects on serotonergic and adrenergic receptors. In healthy volunteers, its effects on D2 receptors reduce prolactin plasma levels, and induce nausea and hypotension. DHEC improves parkinsonian signs in the MPTP-treated monkey model of PD and preclinical data suggest that DHEC may have neuroprotective properties.

In clinical practice, DHEC is used as monotherapy in de-novo PD patients. Bergamasco et al [21] reported significant improvement of motor scores in 123 de-novo PD patients compared to placebo, whereas several smaller trials reported a comparable effect of DHEC and bromocriptine in de-novo PD patients. DHEC is also used as add on therapy in advanced PD patients. In this situation it also appears to be as effective as bromocriptine. Studies comparing DHEC with newer dopamine agonists are lacking. The usual daily dose ranges from 10 to 40 mg t.i.d. with an up titration of 10mg/week. Side effects that have been reported include nausea, hallucinations, orthostatic reactions, and insomnia. Retroperitoneal or pleural fibrosis, which has been described with all other ergot dopamine agonists, has not been reported so far in DHEC treated patients [22].

PIRIBEDIL is a non-ergot D2/D-3 agonist with alpha-2 antagonistic effects. Piribedil is effective in reversing parkinsonian symptoms in the MPTP-treated primate. There is also some evidence that piribedil has neuroprotective effects in experimental models.

Piribedil is administered orally. T_{max} is reached within one hour and it has a relatively long plasma elimination half-life of 20 hours. Piribedil solubility allows it to be used intravenously for experimental purposes or acute challenge tests.

Piribedil is effective either as monotherapy in de-novo PD patients [23] or as an add-on to preexisting levodopa therapy [24]. Pirebedil is given as 50 mg tablets, with a starting dose of 50 mg/day, increasing every two weeks in 50 mg increments to a usual maximum dose of 150 mg/day. Adverse events associated with pirebedil treatment are similar to those reported with other dopamine agonists including gastrointestinal, cardiovascular, and neuropsychiatric events.

APOMORPHINE is a potent dopamine agonist with high affinity to D_1 and D_2 receptors. When given orally, apomorphine is a nearly completely cleared by first pass hepatic metabolism. Therefore, apomorphine is administered by alternative routes, including subcutaneous injection. Because of its lipophilic character, it equilibrates rapidly from peripheral to central compartments.

The elimination half-life is about 30 minutes. Its main metabolic route is auto-oxidation and excretion by the liver, with only about 3-4% excreted unchanged in the urine.

How can Apomorphine be delivered in continuous fashion?

Apomorphine is licensed in both the US and Europe as a "rescue" medication to reverse OFF-periods in fluctuating PD patients. For this indication, it is administered "on demand" as single subcutaneous injections via pen injectors. This apomorphine pen (APO-go pen®) is a prefilled penject device in the form of a pencil. The individual injection dose can be fixed. Usually a pen contains 3 ml of apomorphine (30 mg). After an injection, the needle has to be withdrawn and before the next use, a new one has to put on the pen. The expiry time is 48 hours after the first needle has been attached.

The main advantage of rescue apomorphine injections is the very fast onset of effect compared to oral dopaminergic drugs. This effect is independent of gastrointestinal factors, such as prior ingestion of food. The onset of clinical effect is in about 10 minutes, and the duration of effect lasts up to 60-90 minutes. The apomorphine dose used for a single injection must be evaluated for each patient individually by an apomorphine challenge test (see below). Usual doses ranges from 3 to 6mg per injection.

In Europe, apomorphine is also used as a means to achieve continuous dopaminergic drug delivery in patients with refractory ON-OFF oscillations. Continuous subcutaneous infusions of apomorphine were pioneered by Lees and co-workers in the 1980's [25] and are now licensed in Europe under the trade name of "APO–go®". The Crono APO-go syringe driver is a small portable device with a 10 or 20 ml syringe and an infusion catheter attached. It can be carried hidden under a shirt. The needle of the infusion catheter is fixed subcutaneously, usually in the abdominal wall. The pump allows an adjustment of the dose rate and additional bolus injections as required. The system includes a display, which informs the patient how much longer the infusion will run. Depending on the daily dose, the syringe and the infusion catheter have to be changed once or twice every 24 hours.

What is the indication for a continuous subcutaneous apomorphine pump?

The continuous subcutaneous administration of apomorphine via pump provides a sustained level of dopamine receptor stimulation. Therefore, the therapy is used in PD patients with a good response to levodopa but who experience motor fluctuations with prolonged, frequent, or unpredictable "off" periods despite an optimal oral medication regimen [26, 27]. It can be used as an add-on to continuing oral therapy or alone as monotherapy. The infusion normally runs during the patient's waking day, however, some patients require 24-hour administration, often with a lower infusion rate during the night. Clinical studies report a reduction of daily off time of 40 to 80% with daily doses of apomorphine between 30 and 150 mg/day. The daily levodopa dose requirement can usually be reduced by about 50 - 60% with some patients switching completely to subcutaneous apomorphine alone. Pre-existing levodopa-induced dyskinesias can also be successfully reduced or sometimes abolished by switching to continuous subcutaneous apomorphine infusions [28].

What are the side effects of continuous subcutaneous apomorphine infusion therapy?

The most common side effect of apomorphine administration is nausea. It occurs in about 15% of patients and can usually be counteracted successfully with domperidone. Especially at the start of apomorphine continuous infusions, pre-existing dyskinesias may worsen, thereby requiring dose adjustments. Other side effects include hypotension, confusion, hallucinations, psychosis, eosinophilia, sedation, sleep attacks and sometimes increased libido. Induration and subcutanious nodules may appear at infusion sites. These nodules are often asymptomatic but they can reduce apomorphine absorption. Infections or skin necrosis at infusion sites are rare and usually require a discontinuation of therapy. A rare but serious side effect is the appearance of a Coombs positive autoimmune-hemolytic anemia. The anemia is reversible after discontinuing apomorphine therapy [29]. Therefore, blood counts, haptoglobin, and Coombs test should be evaluated regularly in every patient receiving apomorphine continuous infusion therapy.

What is an apomorphine challenge?

Apomorphine challenge tests are used as a diagnostic tool to assess
dopaminergic responsiveness in parkinsonian patients. Hughes et al[30] reported
a meta-analysis of eight studies with apomorphine challenges and found that
this test had a positive predictive value of 93% and a negative predictive value
of 73% for a diagnosis of Parkinson's disease in a group of patients with
different parkinsonian syndromes. However, in a group of de-novo parkinsonian
patients, the negative predictive value was only 60%. This means that a positive
apomorphine challenge test supports a diagnosis of Parkinson's disease and
predicts responsiveness to oral dopaminergic therapy, but a negative
apomorphine test in early patients does not exclude PD or subsequent
responsiveness to oral therapy. Pinter et al [31] also described a correlation
between a positive apomorphine challenge and a good outcome after STN DBS
in Parkinson's disease patients.

To perform the test, patients receive pre-treatment with domperidone 24 to 48
hours and one hour prior to the challenge (in order to reduce nausea). The
patient is then tested in the off medication state, usually not having taken PD
medications overnight. A motor examination is then undertaken, typically using
the UPDRS motor exam or other tests such as the hand/arm test or a walking
test. The patient then receives apomorpine as a subcutaneous injection at a
starter dose of 2 mg. The dose is the increased in 1-2 mg increments every 45
minutes until the best motor response is achieved. The motor examination is
then repeated. An apomorphine challenge test is considered positive when the
UPDRS or other motor score is reduced (improved) by at least 20%.

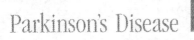

CHAPTER 10

SURGERY FOR PARKINSON'S DISEASE

Kelly E. Lyons, Rajesh Pahwa

What types of surgery are available for patients with Parkinson's disease?

There are two types of surgery widely available for patients with PD[1, 2]. These include creating a lesion in the brain and deep brain stimulation (DBS). Lesion surgeries involve destroying a small target area in the brain. This is usually done by introducing an electrode into the brain with the tip either in the thalamus, globus pallidus interna (GPi) or subthalamic nucleus (STN). The lesions are usually created by heating the electrode tip for approximately one minute. If a lesion is made in the thalamus the procedure is called thalamotomy, in the GPi it is called pallidotomy and in the STN it is called subthalamotomy.

An alternative to creating a lesion is stimulation of a target area (Deep Brain Stimulation). A DBS lead with four contacts is placed into the target area in the brain. The lead is connected by an extension wire that runs down the neck under the skin to an implantable pulse generator (IPG) placed below the collarbone. The IPG is the power supply for the system. When the device is turned on, the electrical current is activated and this modifies firing of neurons in the target site.

There are two kinds of DBS leads available. The intracranial portion of the DBS lead has four contacts, each of which are 1.5 mm in length. One type of lead has contacts separated by 1.5 mm (Model 3387, Medtronic, Inc, Minneapolis, MN) and the other has contacts separated by 0.5 mm (Model 3389, Medtronic Inc, Minneapolis, MN). There are also two kinds of IPGs available, Soletra® and Kinetra®. The Kinetra® stimulator can be connected to two leads for patients who have undergone DBS procedures on both sides of the brain rather than having one IPG (Soletra®) for each side.

The IPGs can be programmed for monopolar stimulation (one of the four electrodes are turned on) or bipolar (two to four electrodes are turned on) stimulation. Using a hand held computer programmer that is placed on the skin over the IPG, the pulse width, amplitude, and frequency of the electric current generated and the choice of active lead contacts can be adjusted. By using a magnet or Access Review Controller® the patient can turn the device on or off. The Access Review Controller® also indicates if the stimulator is on or off. There are different Access Review Controllers used for Soletra® and Kinetra®. The usual stimulation parameters are frequency of 135 to 185 Hz, pulse width of 60 to 120 microseconds and amplitude of 1 to 3 volts[3]. If the electrode tip is in the thalamus it is called thalamic stimulation, in the globus pallidus it is called pallidal stimulation and in the subthalamic nucleus it is called subthalamic stimulation.

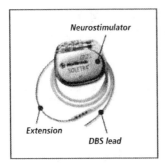

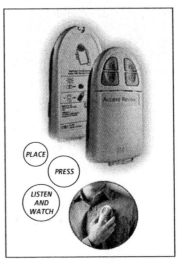

Figure 10.1. *IPG, Lead and extension, (Medtronic, Inc.)*

Figure 10.2. *Access Review Controller® (Medtronic, Inc.)*

How long have surgical therapies been used for Parkinson's disease?

Surgery for PD has been attempted since the start of the 20th century[1]. The modern form of surgery using stereotactic procedures was introduced in the 1940s[4]. Stereotactic procedures involve placement of an electrode or probe in the brain using a brain atlas for reference along with neuroimaging for precise targeting. When this form of surgery was initially introduced, the neuroimaging technique used was ventriculography. Presently, either computerized tomography (CT) or more commonly magnetic resonance imaging (MRI) of the brain are the neuroimaging techniques most often employed[5].

Different targets in the brain were explored to find the best area to improve symptoms with the fewest complications. In 1954, lesions were created in the thalamus to control parkinsonian tremor[6]. Stereotactic surgery gained wide recognition and in 1960, when Leksell and his team observed that posteroventral pallidotomy helped the cardinal symptoms of PD including tremor, bradykinesia and rigidity[7]. The widespread use of surgery for PD was initially limited by the associated morbidity and mortality. With the introduction of levodopa in 1967, there was a rapid decline in the use of these procedures until their resurgence in the late 1980s.

Why is surgical therapy being increasingly used for PD?

The limitations of medical therapy for PD are the major reason for the development of new surgical techniques. When levodopa was initially introduced in 1967 it resulted in marked improvement in symptoms with an associated reduction in morbidity and mortality. However, it was found that with long-term use of levodopa, patients developed motor fluctuations and dyskinesia and in some patients these symptoms resulted in marked disability. In addition, physicians gained a better understanding of the basal ganglia circuitry and a better understanding of the possible surgical targets for PD. Improved neuroimaging and electrophysiological recording techniques led to greater accuracy of the lesions and resulted in reduced morbidity and mortality associated with these surgeries[2].

What does the basal ganglia motor circuitry tell us about the possible targets for PD surgery?

The basal ganglia are made up of different nuclei. The main nuclei of the basal ganglia include the caudate, putamen, and globus pallidus, and clinicians include the STN and the substantia nigra. The basal ganglia have connections to the cortex, brain stem nuclei and the thalamus, which affect movement. The main pathology in PD is in the substantia nigra, which has connections to the striatum (caudate and putamen together are known as the striatum)[8].

The striatum receives excitatory input from the cortex. In addition, it receives excitatory and inhibitory inputs from the substantia nigra. Striatal output is directed to the medial globus pallidus through two pathways, a direct and indirect pathway. The direct pathway involves inhibitory input to the GPi. The indirect pathway involves inhibitory input to the globus pallidus externa, which then sends inhibitory input to the STN, which in turn sends excitatory input to the GPi. The GPi sends inhibitory input to the thalamus, which sends excitatory input to the cortex[8].

In PD, there is loss of substantia nigra neurons and consequently, dopamine in the striatum is reduced. Decreased striatal dopamine diminishes inhibition of the GPi via the direct pathway and increases stimulation of the GPi via the indirect pathway (figure 3, 4). GPi and STN are both overactive in PD. There is increased inhibition of the thalamocortical pathway by the GPi, which in turn leads to reduced output from the motor cortex. Reduced output from the motor cortex manifests as signs of PD, namely bradykinesia and rigidity[8].

In PD, a lesion of the GPi would abolish over-firing of the GPi, eliminate the increased inhibition of the thalamocortical pathway and normalize output from the motor cortex (figure 3). This could lead to improvement of bradykinesia and rigidity. Similarly, the STN is also overactive in PD and an STN lesion would reduce over-stimulation of the GPi via the indirect pathway (figure 4)[8].

In general, which PD patients are candidates for surgery?

PD patients who respond to levodopa and have motor fluctuations and/or dyskinesia that cannot be controlled with medications and patients with disabling tremor that cannot be controlled with medications are candidates for surgery. Patients should not have dementia, behavioral, or psychiatric problems. Patients with other medical conditions that would increase the risk of surgery and patients with atypical parkinsonism are not candidates for these surgeries.

What tests are done to determine an appropriate candidate for these procedures?

One needs to undergo evaluation with a neurologist with expertise in surgical therapy for PD. The benefit from surgery is dependent on a correct diagnosis of PD. The neurologist will confirm the diagnosis of PD and rule out atypical parkinsonism or other causes of parkinsonian symptoms.

A levodopa challenge to determine the patient's response to levodopa is generally performed for patients undergoing evaluation for GPi or STN stimulation. The levodopa challenge involves evaluation of the patient after PD medications are withheld overnight for approximately twelve hours (medication off state) and re-evaluation after the usual morning PD medications are given,

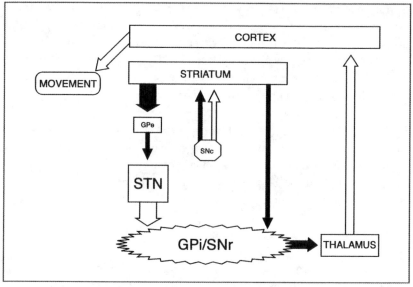

Figure 10.3. *Schematic representation of the effect of pallidotomy. Overfiring of the GPi and resultant excessive inhibition of the thalamocortical pathway are returned toward normal. See text for details.*

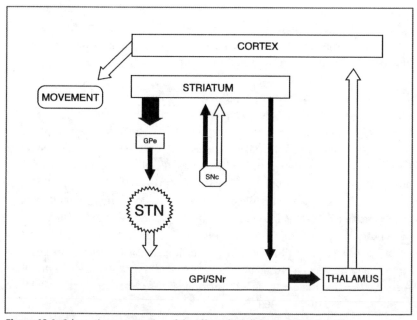

Figure 10.4. *Schematic representation of the effect of subthalamic nucleus lesioning. STN-driven over-firing of the GPi and resultant excessive inhibition of the thalamocortical pathway are returned toward normal.*

or in some cases after a dose of levodopa higher than the usual dose, (medication on state) to determine the extent of the response to levodopa. This helps predict the possible improvement that can be expected from surgery. A patient that does not respond to levodopa will most likely not get a good response from surgery. An MRI of the head is also performed to be sure that there are no significant abnormalities that might affect the outcome of the surgery.

Finally, neuropsychological testing, in most cases a complete battery that takes approximately two to four hours, is performed to determine if there are any significant memory, behavioral, or cognitive problems. Other routine preoperative tests such as blood work and electrocardiogram (EKG), are performed by the neurosurgeon and the anesthesiologist.

How is lesion surgery performed?

On the day of the surgery the patient is admitted to the hospital in the medication off state. The neurosurgeon usually begins the procedure by attaching a stereotactic frame (a halo-type device) to the patient's head. There are different kinds of frames available. The function of the frame is to stabilize the head during surgery so that it is immobilized and to help the neurosurgeon determine the precise area to target for surgery. To attach the frame, the surgeon uses local anesthesia on four areas around the head and the frame is then attached by four screws to the outer part of the skull [5, 9].

Some surgeons have started using a frameless system in which fiducial markers (tiny screws) are attached to the scalp under local anesthesia before neuroimaging is performed. Neuroimaging can then be done as an outpatient procedure rather than on the day of surgery [10]. Once the patient has undergone either a CT, or more often, an MRI of the head, the neurosurgeon uses a brain atlas along with images from the CT or the MRI to determine the exact distances to the target nuclei (thalamus, GPi or STN) and how deep and in what direction the electrode needs to go into the brain. The targeting takes approximately 30 minutes. An area on the top of the head is cleaned and shaved. Local anesthesia is injected for the incision. An incision approximately two inches long is made and then a drill is used to make a hole in the skull the size of a nickel. A system to guide the electrode into the brain is then attached to the head frame or the frameless system is used [5, 9].

Most neurosurgeons use a technique called microelectrode recording to help locate the precise target area. This technique is used in addition to the initial mapping and targeting. Microelectrode recording is a technique where a special electrode is passed into the brain. This electrode detects and measures nearby electrical impulses to help the physician locate the electrode tip. Different target areas can be identified by their unique electrical firing patterns. This process can take approximately two hours [5, 9].

Once the targeted area is identified, a thermocouple electrode is placed in the brain. Initially the electrode is electrically stimulated to assess for any abnormal sensations or movements, such as muscle spasms. For lesion surgeries, if no abnormal sensations or movements occur and benefit is apparent, the lesion is created by heating the tip of the electrode for approximately one minute. This destroys the cells at the tip of the electrode. The electrode is then removed and the skin incision is sutured and the frame is taken off. General anesthesia is not used for this procedure and the patient is awake during the surgery [9].

What are the different types of lesion surgery?

Thalamotomy, pallidotomy and subthalamotomy are the three lesion surgeries for PD. Thalamotomy involves creating a lesion in the ventral intermediate (VIM) nucleus of the thalamus and is used most commonly for essential tremor. In PD, it is rarely used, as it is reserved for patients with disabling medication resistant tremor as the primary symptom and minimal to no disability from other parkinsonian symptoms. Thalamotomy has been reported to improve tremor on the side opposite the surgery in more than 90% of patients with little to no effect on other parkinsonian symptoms [1]. The improvement in tremor has shown to be maintained for up to 11 years after the surgery [11-14]. Thalamotomy has now largely been replaced by DBS of the VIM nucleus of the thalamus.

Pallidotomy involves creating a lesion in the GPi and has been the most commonly performed lesion surgery for PD. Unlike thalamotomy, pallidotomy provides improvement for all cardinal symptoms of PD; tremor, rigidity and bradykinesia as well as a reduction in dyskinesia [15]. Pallidotomy is an option in patients who are responsive to levodopa and have disabling medication resistant motor fluctuations and/or dyskinesia. In a review of the literature, the average improvement in motor scores in the medication off state was 45% and the reduction in dyskinesia on the side opposite of the surgery was 86% [15]. Long-term benefits of pallidotomy have been shown; however, benefits were reduced over time as the disease progressed and additional surgeries were necessary in some patients [16-18]. Pallidotomy has now largely been replaced by DBS of the GPi or STN.

Subthalamotomy involves creating a lesion in the STN and to date is rarely performed in the United States. However, due to the cost of DBS hardware, there is interest in this procedure, especially in less developed countries. In an open label study of 18 patients, subthalamotomy was shown to significantly improve the cardinal symptoms of PD, as well as dyskinesia and allowed a significant reduction in levodopa. These effects were shown to persist for up to three years [19, 20].

How was deep brain stimulation developed?

During lesioning procedures, high frequency stimulation is used to assess improvement in symptoms and any adverse effects before creating the lesion. It had been established that patients with bilateral lesions had a relatively high risk of complications, particularly speech and balance difficulty [21-23]. Benabid and colleagues [24] proposed that instead of creating a lesion, using chronic stimulation could be an option and if patients had significant adverse effects, the stimulation could be reduced or discontinued. Initial studies were promising and DBS became an option for clinical use.

Why has DBS largely replaced lesion surgeries for PD?

The main advantages of DBS surgery are that it is adjustable and reversible. The electrical stimulation parameters can be adjusted to improve symptoms or reduce side effects. DBS does not damage the brain and hence if there are future therapies that can slow disease progression or cure the disease such therapies could still be used. Lesion surgeries are only adjustable by making an additional or larger lesion in the brain and the part of the brain that is lesioned is destroyed, so future therapies acting on that part of the brain might not be an option. In addition, there is a relatively high risk of speech and balance problems after bilateral lesion surgery; however, with bilateral DBS, if these symptoms occur the stimulation can be reduced or discontinued if necessary.

The disadvantages of DBS include the cost of the system and the time and effort involved in programming the stimulator, which requires multiple visits to the surgical center. Patients may also need to undergo repeat surgeries due to device related problems and IPGs are generally replaced every 3-5 years [1].

How is deep brain stimulation surgery performed?

The initial procedure is similar to that previously described for lesion surgery. Once the target has been localized with the help of microelectrode recordings, rather than heating the electrode tip to create a lesion, the DBS electrode is implanted into the brain. Test stimulation is performed to assess for benefit and any abnormal sensations, movements, or side effects. If there is an appropriate response, the electrode is secured to the skull. If the patient is having bilateral procedures performed, the surgery is repeated on the second side either on the same day (simultaneous bilateral procedure) or at a later time (staged bilateral procedure). Once both electrodes are secured to the skull, the incision is sutured and the frame is removed [5].

The second phase of the surgery is usually done approximately one week later. This portion is the only part of the surgery that is performed under general anesthesia. During this procedure, the extension wire, which is connected to the DBS lead is tunneled under the skin down the neck and an incision is made below the collar bone where the IPG is connected to the extension wire. Both incisions are sutured and the procedure is repeated on the second side for bilateral procedures [5].

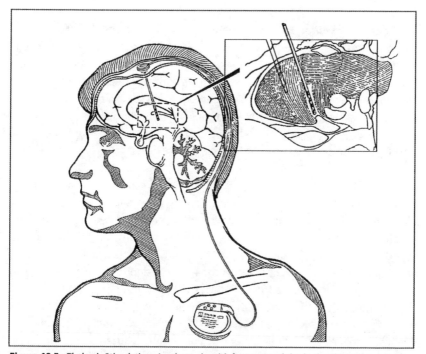

Figure 10.5. *Thalamic Stimulation. An electrode with four exposed tips is placed into the ventral intermediate (VIM) nucleus of the thalamus. The electrode is attached to an extension wire that runs beneath the skin to the implantable pulse generator (IPG) placed in the chest wall (this procedure is similar for pallidal and subthalamic stimulation).*

How does DBS work?

The exact way that DBS works is unknown. As the benefits of DBS are similar to those observed after creating lesions in the thalamus, GPi and STN, it has been proposed that DBS works by reducing the over-activity in these nuclei. The other possibility is that the electrical discharges from these nuclei become abnormal and irregular in patients with PD and DBS resets the electrical discharges and makes them more regular [25].

What are the types of DBS used in PD?

Stimulation of the VIM nucleus of the thalamus, globus pallidus interna (GPi), and subthalamic nucleus (STN) can be performed for PD. The most common surgical procedure for PD is DBS of the STN [2].

Which patients are candidates for thalamic stimulation?

Thalamic stimulation is recommended for tremor predominant patients who have disabling medication resistant tremor. These patients should have minimal signs of bradykinesia and rigidity, as these symptoms are not improved with thalamic stimulation. In addition, patients should not have any significant memory, behavioral, or psychiatric problems, or other unstable medical diagnoses that may increase the risk of surgery. Patients with a combination of PD tremor and essential tremor are also candidates for this surgery.

What are the benefits of thalamic stimulation?

The majority of studies have reported that tremor is markedly improved with thalamic stimulation [26-32]. However, this often does not result in significant improvements in activities of daily living, such as feeding, dressing and tasks involving daily hygiene due to the lack of improvement in bradykinesia, rigidity, and dyskinesia. A double-blind, multi-center study in 24 PD patients who had undergone unilateral thalamic stimulation reported significant tremor improvement at one year, although activities of daily living were not significantly changed [30]. Another multi-center trial with 57 PD patients who had undergone unilateral implants and 16 PD patients who had undergone bilateral implants [31] reported tremor was significantly reduced at one year by 74%. Another study reported 19 PD patients who demonstrated an 82% reduction in tremor on the side opposite the surgery [32]. However, there was no improvement in activities of daily living or other aspects of PD.

What are the long-term benefits of thalamic stimulation?

Pollak and colleagues[26] reported 80 PD patients who had thalamic stimulation for medication-resistant tremor. Tremor remained under good control at an average follow-up of three years with a maximum follow-up of seven years. There was no dramatic effect on other symptoms, including bradykinesia, rigidity or dyskinesia. Lyons et al. [33] reported nine PD patients who were followed for an average of 40 months. Although tremor scores continued to be significantly improved (87%) patients had worsening of bradykinesia, rigidity, and gait due to progression of the disease. Rehncrona et al. [34] reported 20 PD patients followed for six to seven years after thalamic DBS. Tremor continued to be improved; however, there was an overall worsening due to the progression of other PD symptoms.

What patients are candidates for GPi stimulation?

Patients with levodopa responsive PD who have disabling motor fluctuations or dyskinesia may be candidates for GPi stimulation. Patients should not have significant memory, behavioral, or psychiatric problems, or any other medical condition that may increase the risk of surgery.

What are the benefits of GPi stimulation?

GPi stimulation has been shown to improve tremor, bradykinesia, and rigidity, and markedly reduce levodopa-induced dyskinesia. The improvement in parkinsonian symptoms in the medication off state has been reported to be from 27 to 80% with the largest improvements for tremor[35-39]. Improvements in activities of daily living have ranged from 19% to 68%. Improvement in on medication scores has not been consistent and some studies have reported a worsening. All studies reported a significant reduction in dyskinesia resulting in an increase in on time without dyskinesia during the day.

Most of the studies of GPi stimulation have evaluated a small series of patients; however, a multi-center, multinational study of bilateral GPi stimulation reported results from 41 PD patients[37]. Thirty-eight patients were implanted as two patients had cerebral hemorrhage and one patient had intraoperative confusion. In the off medication state, all cardinal features of PD improved; tremor improved by 59%, rigidity by 31%, bradykinesia by 26%, gait by 35% and postural instability by 36%. Patient diaries revealed that the percentage of on time without dyskinesia increased from 28 to 64% and off time was reduced from 37 to 24%. The mean dose of antiparkinsonian medications was unchanged at six months.

What are the long term benefits of GPi stimulation?

There are only a few long-term follow-up studies of GPi stimulation. Ghika et al [38] reported six PD patients with a minimum follow-up of 24 months. Although improvements persisted beyond two years after surgery, signs of decreased efficacy were seen after 12 months. Another report evaluated six patients for approximately three years [40]. Dyskinesia severity and activities of daily living continued to be significantly improved. However, improvement in mean daily duration of off time was lost at the last assessment. Another study examined nine PD patients an average of 48.5 months after GPi stimulation [41]. These investigators reported a 37% improvement in motor function compared to baseline and an increase in on time from 25% of the day at baseline to 59% at the longest follow-up.

Which patients are candidates for STN stimulation?

Patients with levodopa responsive PD who have motor fluctuations and dyskinesia that cannot be improved by medication adjustments are candidates for this procedure. Patients should not have memory, behavioral, or psychiatric problems such as severe depression. In addition, patients should not have any other medical condition that would increase the risk of surgery.

What are the benefits of STN stimulation?

There are multiple reports of the antiparkinsonian effects of STN stimulation [37, 42-46]. Reports have noted improvements in all motor symptoms of PD including tremor, rigidity, bradykinesia, posture, and gait in the medication off state. There is marked improvement in dyskinesia due to reduction in antiparkinsonian medications after surgery and improvement in the duration of on time. Improvement in activities of daily living has ranged from 30-72% and motor score improvements have ranged from 42-74% in the off medication state. Anti-parkinsonian medications are usually reduced by 37-80% after surgery, resulting in a 63-81% reduction in dyskinesia.

One of the largest studies of bilateral STN stimulation is a multi-center, multinational study of 96 PD patients [37]. In the off medication state there was a mean improvement of 44% in activities of daily living and a mean improvement of 51% in motor scores. All motor subscores in the off medication state also improved; tremor by 79%, rigidity by 58%, bradykinesia by 42%, gait by 56%, and postural instability by 50%. Patient home diaries revealed a reduction in off time of 61%, an increase in on time of 64%, and a decrease in on time with dyskinesia of 70%.

What are the long-term benefits of STN stimulation?

Multiple studies have examined the long-term benefits of STN stimulation [47-50]. Pahwa et al [48] reported 19 PD patients after up to 42 months follow-up. Significant improvements in activities of daily living and motor function were maintained, on time was increased from 38% at baseline to 72%, off time was reduced from 43% to 17%, anti-parkinsonian medications were reduced 57%, and dyskinesia was reduced 42%. Similar results were found by Kleiner-Fisman et al [49] in 25 PD patients after 30 months of follow-up. Krack et al [50] followed 49 PD patients five years after bilateral STN. They reported a 49% improvement in activities of daily living, a 54% improvement in motor function, a 71% reduction in dyskinesia, and a 63% reduction in anti-parkinsonian medication compared to baseline. However, PD did continue to progress and worsening of axial symptoms as well as the development of dementia did occur.

Is bilateral STN stimulation superior to bilateral GPi stimulation?

Although the criteria for patient selection for GPi and STN stimulation are similar, there are several small studies [44, 51-54] but no large studies that have randomly compared these two procedures. Krack et al [44] compared eight PD patients who underwent STN stimulation and five PD patients who underwent GPi. After six months of follow-up, motor scores were improved 71% with STN stimulation and 39% with GPi stimulation. Improvements in rigidity and tremor were comparable but more improvement in bradykinesia was seen with STN stimulation. In addition, there was a reduction in levodopa dosage only in the STN group.

Burchiel et al. [51] performed a randomized study in 10 PD patients with five patients undergoing GPi and five undergoing STN stimulation. At 12 months there was a similar improvement in both groups but only patients in the STN group had a reduction in anti-parkinsonian medications. Volkmann et al. [52] reported a 54% improvement in parkinsonian signs with GPi stimulation as compared to a 67% improvement with STN stimulation, and medication was reduced only in the STN group. Krause et al. [54] also compared GPi and STN stimulation and found that only the STN group had improvements in activities of daily living and motor function; however, both groups had a reduction in dyskinesia. As demonstrated in these studies, STN stimulation appears to provide greater benefit compared to GPi stimulation and is currently the surgical treatment of choice for PD.

Do any factors predict the outcome of DBS?

Predictive factors for outcome from DBS have only been examined for STN DBS. Welter et al. [55] examined predictors of outcome in 41 PD patients. They found that younger age, shorter disease duration, and a positive response to levodopa (levodopa challenge response) were the best predictors of outcome. Charles et al. [56] and Jaggi et al. [57] reported that younger age and preoperative response to levodopa were the strongest predictors of STN DBS outcome.

Kleiner-Fisman et al. [49] examined 25 patients and Pahwa et al. [58] examined 45 patients and both found that the preoperative response to levodopa was the strongest predictor of outcome after STN DBS. Given the results of these studies, the magnitude of the response to levodopa preoperatively is the strongest predictor of STN DBS outcome; however, age may also have an impact on outcome with younger patients tending to do better than older patients.

What are the risks of DBS surgery?

Side effects of DBS are similar for the three targets (thalamic, GPi, and STN) and can be divided into those related to the surgical procedure, those associated with the device, and those associated with stimulation. These complications are to some extent dependent on the expertise of the neurosurgeon, patient selection, and mechanical problems associated with the devices. Several papers have reported large series of patients, specifically examining complications due to DBS [59-62]. The findings of these studies have been combined to include 360 patients receiving DBS of which 288 were PD patients.

Surgical Complications
Surgical complications usually occur within 30 days of surgery. These complications are similar to those from other types of brain surgery and usually occur in less than 5% of patients. These complications include intracranial bleeds, strokes, seizures, infections, lead misplacement, and death. In 360 patients reported [59-62], death occurred in two patients (pulmonary embolism and

aspiration pneumonia) representing 0.6% of patients. Complications resulting in permanent neurological deficits occurred in 2.8% of the patients. Surgical complications without permanent neurological deficit included infection (5.6%), hemorrhage (3.1%), disorientation (2.8%), lead reposition due to misplacement (2.8%), seizures (1.1%), pulmonary embolism (0.6%), cerebral spinal fluid leak (0.6%), peripheral nerve injury (0.6%) and venous infarction (0.3%).

Device Related Complications

Device-related complications refer to those related directly to the functioning of the hardware of the system including the lead, extension wire, and IPG. These complications generally require additional surgery to replace the malfunctioning part of the system. Device related complications have been shown to occur in approximately 25% of patients receiving DBS[60, 62]. In 360 patients reported[59-62] lead replacements due to migration, fracture, or malfunction occurred in 5%, replacement of extension wire due to fracture or erosion occurred in 4.4%, IPG malfunction occurred in 4.2%, IPG repositioning due to pain, tissue growth, or for cosmetic purposes occurred in 1.7%, and apparent allergic reactions to the system occurred in 0.6%. Although it is not considered a complication, battery replacement, which requires an additional outpatient surgery, occurs approximately every three to five years depending upon stimulation parameters used.

Stimulation Related Complications

Side effects related to stimulation depend on the exact location of the tip of the lead and the intensity of stimulation. The majority of these side effects can be reduced by either using another lead contact or reducing the stimulation intensity. These side effects include eyelid closure, double vision, muscle spasms, tingling, hemiballismus, numbness, speech difficulties, mood changes, depression, increased sexual desire, vision changes, balance difficulties, and pain. Occasionally non-specific sensations such as anxiety, panic, palpitations, and nausea can also occur.

Most often, reducing the stimulation intensity or changing the combination of active lead contacts may reduce the side effects but may also lead to loss of benefit. In some patients, additional surgery may be required to change the location of the lead if it is determined, generally with neuroimaging, that the lead is misplaced. Depression, manic behavior, increased sexual desire, balance difficulties, and speech difficulties can be very bothersome, and some patients may require medications to control these side effects.

Are there any contraindications to DBS?

DBS is contraindicated in patients who have a medical diagnosis that requires MRIs using full body scan or a head transmit coil that extends to the upper chest because of the potential for MRI to cause heating of the leads that could lead to brain damage or damage the stimulator system.

For patients with DBS, diathermy (e.g. short wave diathermy, microwave diathermy, and therapeutic ultrasound diathermy) is contraindicated because the energy can be transmitted to the brain through the extension and leads and can result in brain tissue damage and possibly death. In addition, diathermy can damage the stimulators.

What is the concept of transplantation as a surgical treatment for PD?

Transplantation is an investigational procedure involving the delivery of tissue or other material into an area of the brain. It is hoped that implanted cells can replace the neurons lost due to the disease and hence restore function. This type of procedure is still under investigation and the nature of benefit has varied depending on the kind of material and techniques used for transplantation.

What were the results of adrenal transplantation?

Autologous adrenal medullary transplantation was the first transplant strategy used in PD. The first attempts at adrenal transplantation began in 1982 and resulted in only minimal and transient improvement [63, 64]. However, in 1987, Madrazo et al [65] reported "dramatic amelioration" of symptoms in two young patients. Subsequent investigators noted only modest improvement in function during off time and a mild reduction of off time [66-69]. Most of this benefit was lost by two years [70]. Patients who came to autopsy were found to have few or no surviving transplanted cells [67, 71, 72]. This procedure has now been abandoned.

What were the results of fetal transplantation for PD?

Studies in animal models of PD demonstrated that transplanted fetal mesencephalic neurons survive, form synaptic connections, exhibit normal firing patterns, and improve parkinsonian features [73-77]. These studies also indicated that implantation of appropriate tissue into an appropriate location is necessary for clinical benefit.

Lindvall and coworkers[78] first evaluated fetal grafting in two patients using a mesencephalic cell suspension from single donors. These patients experienced modest but significant improvement in motor function in the off state. Since then, several hundred PD patients received transplanted human mesencephalic tissue, mostly in small, unblinded trials[79-85].

Transplanted patients were mostly those with disability related to motor fluctuations that could not be overcome with additional medication changes. Fetal transplants were prepared as blocks of tissue or suspensions of dissociated cells. Donor age varied from five to 17 weeks post-conception and 3 to 5 fetal nigra were generally transplanted per side into the striatum. Some studies employed immunosuppression while others did not. Many of these studies found that transplanted dopamine neurons survived transplantation and led to motor improvement over several months to years, with reductions in off time, improvement in motor function, decreased dyskinesia, and lowering of levodopa doses.

PET studies showed fluorodopa uptake was increased, thereby suggesting tissue survival[82, 84, 85]. Autopsies performed on two transplanted patients demonstrated healthy graft tissue, including large numbers of surviving dopaminergic cells, and physiologic reinnervation patterns[81]. Thus, evidence from open label studies indicated that transplanted embryonic mesencephalic cells could survive transplantation, at least partially re-innervate the striatum, and take up dopa. In addition, these studies suggested clinical benefit, especially with regard to improving motor function during the off state and decreasing off time. However, any clinical benefit observed in open label studies could potentially be due in part or whole to placebo effects.

What were the results of fetal cell transplantation in double-blind studies?

Freed et al[86] evaluated transplantation of embryonic dopamine neurons into 40 advanced PD patients in a double-blind, sham surgery-controlled trial. Patients (34 to 75 years of age, mean disease duration 14 years) were randomly assigned to undergo transplantation or sham surgery, and were followed in a double-blind manner for one year, after which time those in the sham surgery group were offered transplantation. Mesencephalic tissue from a total of four embryos was transplanted into the putamen bilaterally. All patients had PD for more than seven years, and had a positive response to levodopa. The primary outcome measure was a subjective global rating of change that was mailed in by patients 12 months following surgery. According to this scale, there was not a significant difference between transplanted and non-transplanted groups.

There were no differences in mean global rating scores (0.0 vs. -0.4) and there were no differences in clinical motor function at one year. However, younger patients who were transplanted had a 28% improvement in total Unified Parkinson's Disease Rating Scale (UPDRS) scores compared to the sham surgery group. UPDRS motor scores off medication improved 18% for the whole transplantation group and 34% for the younger patients. 18F-fluorodopa uptake in the putamen on PET increased 40% in the transplanted group compared to a decline of 2% in the sham-surgery group. Autopsy results in two patients who died from causes unrelated to surgery revealed 2,000 to 23,000 surviving transplanted dopamine neurons per transplant track.

In another study [87], 34 advanced PD patients were randomized to receive bilateral transplantation with one donor per side, four donors per side, or sham procedures. Patients were followed for two years and the primary outcome variable was UPDRS motor score in the morning before medication intake. Thirty-one patients completed the trial, and two died during the trial and three afterward, all for causes unrelated to the surgery. Patients who received transplantation with four donors demonstrated very well innervated striata on autopsy. PET results demonstrated a significant dose-dependent increase in fluorodopa uptake with no change in sham surgery patients and an approximate one-third increase in patients receiving four donors. However, no significant differences were identified in clinical measures following transplantation. Increases (worsening) compared to baseline in UPDRS motor scores while off medication were 9.4 for placebo, 3.5 for one donor per side and -0.72 for four donors per side.

Double-blind studies confirm that transplanted fetal mesencephalic cells can survive transplantation as evidenced by both autopsy studies and increased fluorodopa uptake on PET scans. These studies have not demonstrated definitive benefit, although they do suggest modest clinical benefit in various measures of PD severity. Further research is required to determine why such limited clinical benefit is achieved relative to cell survival and apparent striatal reinnervation.

Were there any major side effects from fetal cell transplanttransplantation?

Thirty-three patients in the Freed et al. study[86] ultimately received transplants and were followed for as long as three years after surgery. Dystonia and dyskinesia that persisted after elimination or reduction of antiparkinsonian therapy ("runaway dyskinesia") occurred in five (15%) of the 33 patients more than one year after surgery. In the second study[87], 13 of 23 transplanted patients developed off-medication dyskinesia requiring subsequent DBS. No off medication dyskinesia was observed in sham surgery patients. The cause of the dyskinesia despite discontinuation of medication is poorly understood, but to some extent appears to be related to unregulated or patchy dopamine release from grafts[88].

What were the results of transplantation of porcine (pig) dopamine cells?

Although an open label study suggested possible clinical benefit[89, 90], a subsequent double-blind study[91] did not identify significant improvement comparing transplanted to non-transplanted patients. This experience highlights the fact that a substantial placebo effect can be seen in surgical trials in PD and points to the need for definitive randomized, double-blind, sham surgery controlled studies. Transplantation with porcine cells has been abandoned.

What is the status of human retinal cell transplantation?

Transplanted cultured human retinal pigment epithelial cells (RPE) are currently being evaluated as a source of levodopa and dopamine that may improve parkinsonian symptoms. RPE cells are harvested from the inner layer of the retina between the photoreceptors and choriocapillaris[92], and have been shown to survive in rodent and non-human primate models with minimal host immune response while improving parkinsonian symptoms[93].

Watts et al. evaluated the safety and efficacy of unilateral RPE transplantation in 6 advanced PD patients in an open-label pilot study[94]. RPE cells attached to cross-linked gelatin microcarriers (Spheramine) were implanted into the post-commissural putamen contralateral to the worst affected side and no immunosuppression was used. At 12 months the motor UPDRS scores in the medication off condition improved 41-61% compared to baseline.

In three patients with 18 months follow-up, improvement was 25-58% and in three patients with 24 months follow-up improvement was 33-46% compared to baseline. A large double-blind study is now underway.

What is the status of stem cell transplantation?

The field of stem cell biology is still in its infancy and many hurdles remain to be overcome. The hope is that stem cells will provide an unlimited, self-renewing source of cells that can be transplanted, migrate to areas of injury or degeneration, and replace lost cells by differentiating into the appropriate cell type and integrating into host neuronal circuitry. It has been relatively difficult to achieve a complete and coordinated induction of multi-potent stem cells into a single cell type. In the laboratory, stem cells are exposed to a variety of complex manipulations and exposures to growth factors and other signals to induce differentiation into dopamine neurons [95]. However, following grafting to date, most of these regimens are plagued by a relatively low proportion of resultant dopamine cells or a poor cell survival rate. It seems likely, though, that further refinements to the differentiation and maintenance regimens will improve this situation over time.

What were the results of glial cell line-derived neurotrophic factor (GDNF) studies in PD and what is the current status of GDNF therapy in PD?

An alternative surgical approach to the treatment of PD is the delivery of neurotrophic factors such as GDNF. GDNF has been shown to protect dopamine neurons and cause axonal regeneration leading to improved functioning in non-human mammals [96]. A randomized, double-blind study of GDNF injected into the cerebral ventricles of PD patients found no improvement and resulted in multiple adverse events [97]. Subsequently, Gill and colleagues [98] examined continual infusion of GDNF into the posterior putamen in an open label study of five PD patients. At the one-year follow-up, they reported no serious side effects and improvements in motor function, activities of daily living, and dyskinesia. At the two-year follow-up, they reported a 57% improvement in motor function and a 63% improvement in activities of living with associated improvements in measures of quality of life [99].

Similarly, Slevin et al. [100] reported 24-week results of an open label study of 10 patients that received unilateral intraputaminal infusion of GDNF. They reported a 30% improvement in motor function and the only side effects reported were Lhermitte symptoms (sudden transient electric-like shocks extending down the spine, triggered by flexing the head forward) in two patients.

Given the positive results of the open label studies, a multi-center, double-blind, placebo-controlled study of 34 patients receiving direct infusion of GDNF into the putamen was conducted [101]. There were no differences between the GDNF and placebo groups in the primary outcome variable, UPDRS motor scores, at the six-month follow-up visit. Based on these results and patient safety concerns, the sponsor discontinued the study.

What is gene therapy?

Gene therapy is investigational and involves modifying the ability of human cells at the DNA level to produce molecules or proteins with therapeutic value, such as dopamine or trophic factors. Two methods of delivery have been used; 1) cells can be genetically modified in the laboratory and later transplanted into the host or 2) altered viruses (virus vectors) are used to directly carry the therapeutic genes to the targeted tissue. PD is a good candidate disease for gene therapy as the neuropathological, neurochemical and clinical changes associated with the disease are well studied [102, 103].

What is the status of gene therapy for PD?

There are several gene therapy studies that are beginning or are planned. Feigin and colleagues [104, 105] reported the safety of adeno-associated virus (AAV) delivery of the glutamic acid decarboxylase (GAD) gene, which synthesizes GABA, the primary inhibitory neurotransmitter in the brain. The goal of STN GAD gene transfer is to shift the output from the STN from mostly excitatory to mostly inhibitory to reduce overfiring of the GPi neurons. In an open label study, 12 patients received subthalamic AAV-GAD gene therapy. There were no serious adverse effects related to the study treatment and UPDRS motor scores off medication were improved by 18% at three months, 9.6% at six months and 7.7% at 12 months.

In a rat model of PD, lentiviral vector striatal gene transfer of aromatic amino acid decarboxylase (AADC; converts L-DOPA into dopamine), tyrosine hydroxylase (TH; converts tyrosine into L-DOPA) and GTP-cyclohydrolase 1 (CH1; synthesizes TH cofactor) resulted in sustained transgene expression, increased dopamine, and functional improvement[106]. A human clinical trial has been proposed to examine the lentiviral vector delivery of these three genes, AADC, TH and CH1, into the striatum to reprogram cells to produce dopamine[107]. AV201, an AAV vector containing the gene for human AADC which is delivered directly to the striatum is being studied as a means to restore dopamine and prolong the effect of levodopa[108].

CERE-120 is a gene therapy product that delivers the neurturin (NTN) gene via an AAV delivery system. The NTN gene encodes the NTN protein that helps maintain survival of dopamine-producing neurons. NTN is a member of the same protein family as GDNF and they have similar effects. A study has been initiated to test the safety and preliminary efficacy of CERE-120 in patients[109].

Gene therapy is an investigational therapy, which could be a promising treatment for PD; however, the current trials are very early human studies focusing primarily on safety and tolerability. A great deal more research, including eventual randomized, double-blind, placebo-controlled studies will be necessary to determine if gene therapy is a safe and effective treatment for PD.

CHAPTER 11

FUTURE TREATMENTS FOR PARKINSON'S DISEASE

Jen C. Moller, Wolfgang H. Oertel

Introduction

This chapter summarizes new developments in the symptomatic, neurorestorative, and neuroprotective therapy of PD. The first sections focus on novel symptomatic treatments not taking into account that some of these compounds, such as the adenosine A_{2A} antagonists, may also have neuroprotective properties. In the middle section, experimental treatments such as stem cell therapy, glial cell line-derived neurotrophic factor (GDNF), and gene therapy are described. GDNF possibly fulfills the requirements for becoming both a neurorestorative and a neuroprotective therapy. Finally, in the last section of this chapter possible neuroprotective treatments based on orally administered compounds are presented.

What is the possible future role of the rotigotine patch in the treatment of PD?

Rotigotine is a lipid-soluble, non-ergoline, selective D2 dopamine receptor agonist with marked antiparkinsonian activity in monkeys [1]. Rotigotine CDS (constant delivery system) contains this dopamine agonist in a transdermal delivery system. After transdermal application of rotigotine, the drug reaches the systemic circulation with a lag time of approximately two to three hours. Maximal plasma concentration of rotigotine is achieved 24 hours after patch application. The silicone-based transdermal patch is replaced every day. In healthy volunteers, a stable plasma level was reached after two to three days with no apparent subsequent accumulation or change in clearance. For the treatment of PD, patches containing different doses of rotigotine were evaluated. Apart from two phase II studies [2, 3], two randomized, placebo-controlled, double-blind studies in patients with early PD [4, 5] and two randomized, placebo-controlled, double-blind studies in patients with advanced PD [6] were performed.

The Parkinson Study Group enrolled a total of 242 patients with early PD[4]. Patients were randomly assigned to treatment with patches containing 4.5, 9, 13.5, or 18 mg rotigotine, or placebo. The duration of the double-blind treatment was 11 weeks, and the primary efficacy variable was the change in the sum of UPDRS parts II (ADL subsection) and III (motor subsection). There was a significant improvement for the 13.5 mg and 18 mg groups compared with placebo. The UPDRS II and III sum score was also improved in the 9 mg group, but the magnitude of change did not reach statistical significance. 277 patients with early PD were enrolled in a second trial, the preliminary results of which were summarized in a recent review[5]. This trial duration was 27 weeks, and patients were titrated weekly in 4.5 mg increments to an optimal response or a maximum dose of 13.5 mg/day. More than 90% of patients in the active treatment arm used the patch containing 13.5 mg rotigotine by the end of maintenance. Patients on rotigotine showed a significant improvement in the UPDRS II and III sum score compared with patients in the placebo group.

Preliminary results of the two randomized, placebo-controlled, double-blind studies in patients with advanced PD were reported in another recent review[6]. The change from baseline in "off" time was used as the primary outcome measure in both trials. In the first trial (n=310) no significant differences in "off" time reduction were found between the placebo group and patients treated with 9 mg, 18 mg, and 27 mg patches, respectively, after seven weeks. This result was probably due to a large placebo effect. In the second trial (n=351), however, a significant "off" time reduction was observed between the 18 mg and 27 mg groups and the placebo group after 24 weeks of treatment.

Side effects were generally consistent with effects due to stimulation of central or peripheral dopamine receptors. The most common side effect was an application site-reaction in up to 44% of the rotigotine-treated patients with early PD[6]. However, less than 5% of the patients receiving rotigotine withdrew from the study because of application site reactions. Apart from the transdermal delivery system, a rotigotine nasal spray for the treatment of acute PD symptoms is currently under development.

Rotigotine CDS may be of special interest for the future therapy of PD for two reasons. First, the transdermal route of delivery and the once daily administration is convenient for the patient. It may also avoid problems arising from erratic gastrointestinal absorption. Patients with swallowing disorders or perioperative patients may also benefit from the administration of rotigotine CDS. Second, the pulsatile mode of action of many dopaminergic drugs such as standard levodopa/DDCI formulations probably contributes to the development of late motor complications including motor fluctuations and dyskinesias. The continuous mode of action of rotigotine CDS may delay these motor complications [5] but no prospective data are yet available.

Will adenosine A$_{2A}$ antagonists play a role in the future treatment of PD?

Adenosine A$_{2A}$ receptors are preferentially localized to the dendrites of GABAergic striatal projection neurons belonging to the indirect pathway [7, 8]. Istradefylline, the most extensively studied adenosine A$_{2A}$ antagonist to date, reduced increased extracellular GABA levels in the globus pallidus after intrastriatal 6-OHDA injection in the rat [9]. Several reports in MPTP-treated primates suggested that istradefylline had antiparkinsonian effects while inducing little or no dyskinesia [7, 10, 11]. The precise mode of action of adenosine A$_{2A}$ antagonists is unknown. It is generally assumed that these compounds exert antiparkinsonian activity by attenuating the overactivity of the indirect pathway caused by striatal dopamine depletion [12].

So far, two double-blind, placebo-controlled, proof-of-principle studies have been performed [12, 13]. In the first study, 15 patients with moderate to advanced PD were assigned to a six-week treatment period with istradefylline (n=12) or placebo (n=3) [13]. The dose of istradefylline was gradually increased to 80 mg/day. Motor function was assessed 1) when istradefylline was given alone, 2) when istradefylline was coadministered with suboptimal intravenous levodopa infusions, and 3) when istradefylline was co-administered with optimal intravenous levodopa infusions. The investigators found that istradefylline failed to alter the severity of parkinsonian (and dyskinetic) symptoms in patients when levodopa was not coadministered or when receiving optimal intravenous levodopa infusions. However, istradefylline significantly potentiated the antiparkinsonian action of suboptimal intravenous levodopa infusions by 36%, but with 45% less dyskinesia compared with that induced by the optimal levodopa infusion alone.

In the second study, 83 levodopa-treated PD patients with motor fluctuations and peak-dose dyskinesias were assigned to a treatment with 20 mg istradefylline/day (n=26), 40 mg istradefylline/day (n=28), or placebo (n=29) [12]. Patients in the combined istradefylline groups experienced a significant reduction in "off" time. Severity of dyskinesia remained unchanged, whereas "on" time with dyskinesia was mildly increased.

Istradefylline is a promising drug for the future treatment of PD. It will probably be most useful for the treatment of advanced PD patients. If the results of the two proof-of-principle studies can be confirmed, istradefylline may be administered as an adjunct to levodopa in patients with motor fluctuations while inducing less dyskinesias than the currently available dopaminergic drugs (i.e., dopamine agonists, COMT inhibitors, MAO-B inhibitors). For the time being, the results of phase III trials investigating the efficacy and safety of istradefylline in advanced PD have to be awaited. Trials comparing istradefylline and other PD medications would also be useful.

Are dopamine reuptake inhibitors a promising future option for the therapy of PD?

The potential usefulness of dopamine reuptake inhibitors such as amphetamines and bupropion in the symptomatic treatment of PD has been discussed for a considerable period of time [14, 15]. Dopamine reuptake inhibitors are supposed to increase the intrasynaptic striatal dopamine concentration and thus to improve motor function. The latest results, however, have not been promising. Although the monoamine reuptake inhibitor brasofensine reversed bradykinesia without inducing dyskinesia in MPTP-treated marmosets, no change in patient disability was observed in a small study in eight patients with moderate PD [16, 17]. Likewise, the novel monoamine reuptake inhibitor NS 2330 failed to alter parkinsonian severity or to prolong the duration of the levodopa response in a recent placebo-controlled study in nine patients with advanced PD [18]. These discouraging results may be due to the low number of remaining striatal dopaminergic synapses and a reduced expression of the dopamine transporter in PD [19].

How will sarizotan and other antidyskinetics be used for the treatment of PD in the future?

Several compounds are under investigation that may reduce dyskinesia without worsening parkinsonian symptoms. These include serotonin 5-HT1A agonists, alpha-2 adrenergic antagonists, and AMPA receptor antagonists. Since exogenous levodopa is predominantly decarboxylated in serotonergic terminals in the advanced stages of PD, stimulation of the serotonin 5-HT1A autoreceptor was hypothesized to improve dyskinesia by allowing more physiological intrasynaptic dopamine concentrations [20]. Accordingly, it was shown that the serotonin 5-HT1A agonist sarizotan significantly reduced levodopa-induced dyskinesias in MPTP-treated monkeys [21]. The alpha-2 adrenergic antagonist idazoxan also reduced dyskinesias and, in addition, prolonged the antiparkinsonian action of levodopa in MPTP-lesioned primates [22].

The precise mode of action of the alpha-2 adrenergic antagonists is not known. The AMPA receptor antagonist talimpanel potentiated the antiparkinsonian action of levodopa and simultaneously decreased dyskinesias in MPTP-lesioned monkeys[23]. Similar to adenosine A_{2A} antagonists, AMPA receptor blockade may lead to a lower activity of the indirect pathway in this animal model[13].

So far, only a limited number of clinical trials on the antidyskinetic action of these compounds have been published. In a recent placebo-controlled study the effects of sarizotan in 18 patients with advanced PD were investigated[20]. When given as adjunct to levodopa, sarizotan reduced the severity of dyskinesias and prolonged the duration of the motor response by approximately 40% each. Idazoxan was initially reported to be ineffective for dyskinesias in a 1-week, placebo-controlled crossover study[24]. The effects of idazoxan were again studied in a placebo-controlled study in 18 PD patients[25]. Although idazoxan led to an improvement in the severity of dyskinesias after an acute levodopa challenge, the observed difference did not reach statistical significance. In addition, two patients dropped out due to side effects caused by an increase in sympathetic tone, i.e., tachycardia and hypertonus.

To date, no clinical data have been published on the effects of another alpha-2 adrenergic antagonist, fipamezole, and the AMPA receptor antagonist talimpanel in PD patients. In summary, the results of additional studies have to be awaited before the role of these compounds in the future therapy of PD can be more precisely assessed. The preclinical and clinical data for sarizotan and the preclinical data for talimpanel lend credence to the assumption that these compounds can be successfully used as an adjunct to levodopa in the treatment of advanced PD patients.

What is the potential of transplantation of stem cells for the future therapy of PD?

Two controlled studies on the transplantation of human embryonic or fetal mesencephalic cells in patients with advanced PD have been published[26, 27]. Overall, the results were not encouraging since the primary outcome measures were not met and persistent "off" dyskinesias developed in a substantial proportion of patients. Despite the considerable potential of stem cells for the treatment of PD, it thus remains to be determined whether these cells can provide benefits superior to what has been obtained with the transplantation of differentiated mesencephalic cells[28].

In principle, three types of stem cells can be considered as a potential source of dopaminergic neurons for transplantation: 1) embryonic stem cells, 2) neural stem cells from the fetal or adult brain, and 3) non-neural stem cells from other sources such as bone marrow and umbilical cord [29]. Overall, a considerable number of protocols have been developed to cause these cells to be differentiated in vitro into dopaminergic neurons [28, 29]. Embryonic stem cells have so far been studied most extensively. Initial focus was on the differentiation of mouse embryonic stem cells, but there are now several publications on human embryonic stem cells and their differentiation into dopaminergic neurons [30-35].

Transplantation of some of these dopaminergic neurons into parkinsonian rats yielded rather mediocre results with respect to cell survival and clinical benefit [30, 31, 33, 35]. The most interesting recent experiment was the transplantation of dopaminergic neurons derived from monkey embryonic stem cells into the putamen of MPTP-treated monkeys [36]. Although only 1.3-2.7% of the transplanted dopaminergic neurons survived, transplantation resulted in a significant improvement in parkinsonian scores, especially for posture and motility.

Neural stem cells may represent the preferred source of dopaminergic neurons since they are already committed to a neural lineage. Several protocols for the differentiation of human neural stem cells into dopaminergic neurons have been developed [37-41]. In one study, mesencephalon-derived human neural progenitor cells were treated with fibroblast growth factor 8, GDNF, and forskolin [40]. Transplantation of these pretreated cells resulted in an elevated production of dopamine and the amelioration of behavioral impairment in parkinsonian rats. Still, only a relatively low number of dopaminergic neurons survived, so some experts believe that neural stem cells will not be the optimal cell type for transplantation in PD [28].

Autologous stem cells such as bone marrow cells avoid the ethical concerns associated with the use of embryonic stem cells, but presently only scarce data are available. In one study, human bone marrow stromal cells were differentiated into dopamine-producing neurons, and improved motor function in 6-OHDA-lesioned rats after intrastriatal transplantation [42].

Besides the transplantation of stem cell-derived dopaminergic neurons, one may hypothetically also take advantage of adult neural stem cells that are localized to specific brain areas. Recently, it has been reported that the generation of neural precursor cells is impaired in PD[43]. This observation raises the possibility of pharmacologically stimulating endogenous neural precursor cells, thereby leading to some neurorestoration in PD.

Overall, stem cell therapy represents a very promising approach to the treatment of PD. Its main advantages are probably the reduction of ethical concerns and the availability of a great number of cells compared with the transplantation of embryonic or fetal mesencephalic neurons. However, there are still quite a few obstacles that have to be overcome:

1) Which type of stem cell is best to use for transplantation and what protocol should be applied with respect to differentiation into dopaminergic neurons, transplantation procedure, implantation site, and concurrent immunosuppression?

2) How can possible side effects such as tumor growth or "off" dyskinesias be avoided?

3) Will the transplantation of dopaminergic neurons derived from stem cells provide more clinical benefit than the transplantation of differentiated mesencephalic neurons, currently available drug treatments, or deep brain stimulation[28]? It is likely that at least 10 years of development and evaluation of transplantation of stem cell-derived dopaminergic neurons will occur before they can become part of clinical practice.

Does the transplantation of Spheramine represent a promising tool for the future treatment of PD?

Human retinal pigmental epithelial cells, that are attached to a microcarrier and secrete levodopa, are another potential future treatment. In an open-label study six patients with advanced PD were transplanted contralateral to the more affected side with a total of 325,000 cells[44]. After six months, UPDRS motor scores during "off" significantly improved by 34%, and no "off" dyskinesias were observed. In addition, three patients had lower dyskinesia scores than at baseline, while the dyskinesia scores of the other three patients remained unchanged. Spheramine implantation appeared to be a safe and potentially effective therapy, and a double-blind controlled trial is currently underway.

Spheramine may have some advantages when compared to stem cells. There are no ethical concerns with respect to the use of Spheramine, and the risk of tumor growth is probably very low. However, it still has to be shown that Spheramine leads to a long-term improvement in parkinsonian disability compared with placebo. As with current stem cell approaches, it also remains to be proven that this invasive dopamine replacement therapy provides better clinical benefit than the currently available drug therapies or deep brain stimulation.

How could neurotrophic factors be used for the future treatment of PD?

The most extensively studied and important neurotrophic factor for dopaminergic neurons is GDNF[45]. This neurotrophic factor was shown to have neurorestorative and neuroprotective properties in 6-OHDA- and MPTP-lesioned rodents[46-48]. In parkinsonian primates, similar observations were made[49-51]. In the most recent study, GDNF was chronically administered via intraventricular or putamenal pumps, leading to bilateral increases in nigral dopaminergic neuron cell size, the number of nigral cells expressing tyrosine hydroxylase, and dopamine metabolite levels in the striatum and pallidum. Moreover, GDNF recipients showed a significant and sustained improvement in parkinsonian features, and there were increases in the dopamine level and the number of tyrosine hydroxylase-positive fibers in the striatum on the lesioned side[50].

Several clinical studies have evaluated GDNF in patients with advanced PD[45]. The first study investigated the safety, tolerability, and biological activity of GDNF delivery via an implanted intracerebroventricular catheter[52]. This multi-center, randomized, double-blind, placebo-controlled study compared the effects of monthly intracerebroventricular administration of placebo, 25, 75, 150, 300, and 500-3000 mg GDNF in 50 PD patients for eight months. Motor performance as measured by the UPDRS was not improved at any dose. Nausea and vomiting were common hours to several days after GDNF infusion. Weight loss occurred in the majority of patients receiving infusions of 75 mg or more. In addition, paresthesias, often described as feelings of electric shocks, were frequently reported. The investigators concluded that GDNF was biologically active as evidenced by the wide range of side effects, but failed to improve parkinsonian features. Postmortem examination of one patient showed no evidence of significant regeneration of nigral neurons or intraparenchymal diffusion of the intracerebroventricular GDNF leading to the assumption that the neurotrophic factor did not reach the target tissues[53].

In the most recent published open label study, GDNF was delivered directly into the putamen of five PD patients using a pump [54]. After one year there were no serious clinical side effects, a 39% improvement in the off-medication UPDRS motor score, and a 61% improvement in the UPDRS ADL score. This clinical improvement was accompanied by a 28% increase in dopamine storage capacity as measured by positron emission tomography (PET) after 18 months.

Although the results have not yet been published, a larger double-blind study of intraputamenal GDNF in PD was recently terminated due to lack of observed efficacy and possible safety concerns [55]. Despite these setbacks in clinical development, GDNF remains one of the most promising candidates for neurorestorative or neuroprotective therapy of PD. The optimum mode of GDNF delivery to the brain of PD patients has yet to be determined. The implantation of encapsulated GDNF-producing cells as examined in MPTP-treated monkeys may represent a suitable option for the delivery of this neurotrophic factor to the brain [56]. Such cells can be transplanted without eliciting an immune response, and they can be retrieved in case of capsule breakage or the occurrence of side effects [45].

A recent publication underlined that the duration of GDNF delivery may be crucial for the maintenance of clinical benefit, since the long term overexpression of GDNF caused the down regulation of tyrosine hydroxylase-activity in striatal dopaminergic terminals [57]. Thus, additional basic and clinical research is necessary to determine how GDNF can be used most efficiently for the treatment of PD.

What are the prospects of gene therapy for the treatment of PD?

A general means for the delivery of potential therapeutic agents to the brain is gene therapy using viral vectors to express selected genes in specific brain areas. Accordingly, gene therapy could also be used for the delivery of GDNF to the striatum or substantia nigra. While this technique has already been successfully used in non-human primates [58], the first trial in humans, which is described in more detail here, attempts the expression of the enzyme glutamic acid decarboxylase (GAD) in the subthalamic nucleus [59].

GAD converts the excitatory neurotransmitter glutamate to the inhibitory neurotransmitter GABA. The subthalamic nucleus is part of the indirect pathway that is overactive in PD, and has glutamatergic output neurons. Thus, the STN nucleus is excessively stimulating the GPi (see figure 1-4). The underlying rationale for STN GAD gene transfer is to change the output of STN neurons from excitatory to inhibitory, thereby reducing the overactivity of the indirect pathway.

Using adeno-associated viral vector-mediated gene transfer, GAD was expressed in the excitatory neurons of the subthalamic nucleus in rats[60]. The transduced neurons were electrically stimulated and then produced inhibitory signals associated with GABA release. This phenotypic shift resulted in neuroprotection of nigral neurons and amelioration of parkinsonian behavior. Subsequently, a protocol for the first double-blind, placebo-controlled trial to evaluate the safety and efficacy of subthalamic GAD gene transfer in PD patients was proposed[59]. The patients, who will undergo deep brain stimulation in the subthalamic nucleus in any event, will be randomized to receive either subthalamic GAD gene transfer via recombinant adeno-associated virus or placebo. For the study period of six months, the stimulators will not be turned on. Subsequently, the patients will be rated by blinded investigators and will have the option to decide whether the stimulators should be turned on or not. The hypothesis is that patients in the treatment arm will not require deep brain stimulation. To date, 11 patients have been recruited for this study, and currently there has been no evidence of any treatment-related side effects[45].

The safety requirements for the injection of viral vectors into the brain are high. The viral vector should incorporate large transgenes, but should also be easy to handle and effectively deliver the transgene to numerous target cells without eliciting an immune host response and any in vivo virus replication[61]. So far, lentivirus- or adeno-associated virus-based recombinant vectors seem the most promising tools for in vivo gene therapy of PD. However, safety issues such as the triggering of autoimmune disease, the activation of endogenous pathogenic viruses, insertional mutagenesis, retrieved replication competence through recombination or superinfection with the wild type virus, and the formation of proteinaceous inclusions are not entirely solved. In addition, gene expression should be controllable since the margin between therapeutic efficacy and potentially deleterious side effects may be narrow. Furthermore, it is not known for how long stable gene expression can be achieved by currently available virus-based vectors[61]. If these technical concerns can be overcome, gene therapy will represent a valuable tool for the neurorestorative, neuroprotective, and possibly symptomatic treatment of PD.

Are there any other possible neuroprotective agents?

Thanks to recent advances, particularly in genetic research into the causes of PD, the neurobiology of this complex disorder is slowly being deciphered [62]. Such diverse molecular and cellular processes as proteasomal dysfunction, protein aggregation, mitochondrial dysfunction, excitotoxicity, apoptosis, and inflammation have been implicated in the degeneration of the dopaminergic neurons in PD. Accordingly, the list of putative neuroprotective agents in PD is long and currently includes antioxidant, promitochondrial, anti-excitotoxic, antiapoptotic, and anti-inflammatory compounds as well as possibly protein aggregation inhibitors in the future [63, 55]. The most important results and developments are summarized here.

Antioxidants were suggested to be neuroprotective, since the content of reduced glutathione in the substantia nigra of PD patients is diminished and dopamine metabolism results in free radical production. Thus, in the DATATOP (Deprenyl and tocopherol antioxidant therapy of PD) study 800 de novo PD patients were treated with 10 mg selegiline/day, 2000 I.U. vitamin E (tocopherol)/day, a combination of selegiline and tocopherol, or placebo [64]. While vitamin E was ineffective, the need for levodopa therapy could be delayed by nine months in the selegiline group. Similar results were observed in the SINDEPAR (Sinemet-Deprenyl-Parlodel) study [65]. This effect of selegiline, however, is probably due to its symptomatic antiparkinsonian efficacy rather than to any neuroprotective properties [66].

According to a recently published study, the novel MAO-B inhibitor rasagiline may have some neuroprotective activity [67]. This activity appears to be independent of MAO-B inhibition.

PD is associated with a mitochondrial dysfunction, as a moderate reduction of complex I activity has been found in the substantia nigra of PD patients and the active metabolite of MPTP (1-methyl-4-phenyl-1, 2, 3, 6-tetrahydropyridin) inhibits complex I of the respiratory chain. Since complex I transfers an electron from NADH to coenzyme Q, the putative neuroprotective efficacy of coenzyme Q was examined in 80 de novo PD patients [68]. 1200 mg coenzyme Q/day led to a significant improvement in UPDRS scores compared to placebo. It remains to be seen, however, whether this observation can be confirmed in a larger study and whether a symptomatic effect of coenzyme Q can be excluded.

The majority of nigral neurons in PD probably dies of apoptosis, i.e., programmed cell death[69]. While the precise mechanisms of apoptosis in PD remain to be elucidated, several compounds with antiapoptotic properties in vitro or in animal models have been tested in patients. These include 1) inhibitors of glyceraldehyde-3-phosphatedehydrogenase (GAPDH), 2) the so-called immunophilins, 3) the antibiotic minocycline, and 4) the c-Jun-N-terminal-kinase (JNK) inhibitor CEP-1347. GAPDH plays a role in glucose metabolism, but can tetramerize under certain conditions and induce apoptosis after translocation into the nucleus. The specific GAPDH inhibitor TCH-346 was tested in PD patients, but so far no official results have been made available.

The immunophilins are immunosuppressive compounds such as FK506 or cyclosporine A, for which binding sites were also identified in the brain. The antiapoptotic activity of immunophilins in vitro and in animal models is not completely understood[70]. The compound GPI-1485, which predominantly binds to neuronal receptors and does not cause any relevant immunosuppression ("neuroimmunophilin"), was examined in PD patients. According to preliminary data, no neuroprotective effect was observed[63].

Minocycline is an approved antibiotic with good penetration across the blood-brain barrier and good long-term tolerability, that showed antiapoptotic activity in vitro and in animal models[71]. The antiapoptotic effect is probably due to inhibition of microglial activation and of cytochrome c release from mitochondria. So far, no data on the putative neuroprotective activity of minocycline in PD have been published. CEP-1347 is a JNK inhibitor, the safety and tolerability of which have been tested in a recent pilot study[72]. Currently, the PRECEPT (Parkinson research examination of CEP-1347) trial is underway that examines its effect on the clinical progression of PD over a study period of 24 months.

In vitro studies have suggested a neuroprotective action of dopamine agonists, that could be due to stimulation of the presynaptic autoreceptor and consequent reduced dopamine release and free radical production[73]. In the CALM-PD-SPECT (Comparison of the agonist pramipexole with levodopa on motor complications of PD - SPECT) study 82 de novo PD patients were initially treated either with 1.5 mg pramipexole/day or 300 mg levodopa/day[74]. The decrease in the density of the dopamine transporter after 46 months was significantly attenuated in the pramipexole group compared to the levodopa group. In the REAL-PET (Requip® as early therapy versus L-Dopa - PET) trial 186 de novo PD patients were initially treated either with ropinirole or levodopa[75]. The patients in the ropinirole group showed a significantly lower reduction of 18F-Dopa uptake after two years than the patients in the levodopa group.

Similar results were observed in the PELMOPET (Pergolide versus L-Dopa as monotherapy in early PD-PET) study[76]. These studies are potentially consistent with slower progression of PD when treated with a dopamine agonist compared to levodopa. Since none of these studies included a placebo group, it cannot be determined whether dopamine agonists slowed the reduction of tracer uptake or whether levodopa accelerated its decrease. According to the results of the ELLDOPA (Earlier vs later L-Dopa) trial, the latter seems more likely[77]. Most importantly, it is not clear whether the observed differences in tracer uptake really reflect differences in the number of remaining dopamine neurons or merely changes in expression of the dopamine transporter gene. Thus, at present it cannot be determined whether dopamine agonists have a neuroprotective effect in PD patients or not.

Conclusions

Current clinical research in PD focuses on the development of non-dopaminergic treatments that avoid or ameliorate dopaminergic motor complications and on the development of neurorestorative and neuroprotective therapies. Although current results underline the difficulties encountered in the development of new treatments, the next decade will probably bring tangible improvements in the therapy of PD. If proven neuroprotective treatments become available, neurologists will have to focus on the early diagnosis of PD. Additional clinical research will also likely address the therapy of symptoms that are caused by the death of non-dopaminergic neurons in PD.

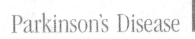

Parkinson's Disease

CHAPTER 12

CASE STUDIES ON PARKINSON'S DISEASE

Mark Stacy

Introduction:

In the initial phase of care for a person with Parkinson's disease, (PD) the diagnosis is of primary importance. Therapeutic discussion and treatment initiation should not begin until both the provider and the patient have similar expectations for benefit. Successful treatment of early Parkinson's disease (PD) is based on correcting primary symptoms of tremor, rigidity, and bradykinesia, while therapy in the moderately advanced population often centers around minimizing motor fluctuations and dyskinesias. Late problems include more severe motor fluctuations and dyskinesias, cognitive dysfunction and hallucinations, falling, bulbar abnormalities, and autonomic disturbances. Depression and anxiety, constipation, and sleep abnormalities can occur during any phase of the disease. Most symptoms can benefit from specific therapeutic interventions, but require good communication between patient and physician.

This section will be divided into case-based illustrations of common issues in managing PD. Specifically, the cases include: Diagnosis of PD, Early Treatment of PD, Treatment of Wearing-Off, Treatment of Dyskinesias, Treatment of Hallucinations, and Treatment of Sleep Difficulty.

1) Diagnosis of Parkinson's Disease:

Patient Description: Jerry is a 58-year-old trucking company owner with a two-year history of walking and balance problems. Although he has not fallen, he must be very careful at work, and tends to lean on furniture when walking at home. He also sometimes has trouble "getting started" when walking and will occasionally stutter-step when in narrow areas. He has noticed a tremor in both hands for at least several years, but his wife remembers his voice "shaking when he gave away [their] daughter" at her wedding more than 10 years ago. The tremor has impaired his ability to work on the farm, and he no longer is able to do his own spot-welding, because he cannot keep the flame steady. He has been seen by another physician who performed an MRI of the brain and neck, EEG, and some blood work. These studies were all normal. He was placed on levodopa and then a dopamine agonist, but they have not made any real difference in his walking or tremor. His wife is frustrated, because Jerry does not seem to be responding to medications like "the books say."

How is Parkinson's Disease Diagnosed?

The diagnosis of PD is based on clinical presentation. A neurologist will check for signs of resting tremor, stiffness or rigidity, and bradykinesia or slowness with rapid movements such as finger tapping or toe tapping. In the case above, the finding of early freezing and balance difficulty is a "red flag" that indicates that Atypical Parkinsonism must be considered in the differential diagnosis. Finally, his tremor, is not resting in nature, and occurs with action (welding) and close questioning finds a much longer history of this symptom. A long history of action tremor suggests the possibility of Essential Tremor.

Are there tests for Parkinson's disease?

The most straightforward patient with PD exhibits the "classic" signs, slowness, stiffness, and resting tremor. Generally, a diagnosis of PD should not be made unless at least two of these three signs are present. Typically, one side is affected more than the other, and patients may also report symptoms of nightmares, sleep difficulty, trouble being heard over the telephone, drooling at night, difficulty turning in bed, trouble cutting food, poor and small handwriting, and a tendency to favor one side.

There are several "red flags" that may prompt a physician to look for other conditions that can resemble the clinical picture of PD. A tremor that is more prominent with action (spilling soup, trouble using a screwdriver or other tools), that has been present for many years, and is also experienced by other family members, strongly suggests a diagnosis of Essential Tremor.

Another clue to the diagnosis of Essential Tremor is a transient reduction in tremor following an alcohol drink, although this does not occur in all cases of Essential Tremor. A lack of resting tremor also prompts investigation into other parkinsonian disorders. Frequent falls and "freezing" at the initial presentation suggests a number of disorders (including PD), and magnetic resonance imaging

(MRI) of the brain is important to exclude vascular parkinsonism (due to multiple strokes) and Normal Pressure hydrocephalus. Furthermore, lack of response to levodopa should be cause to reconsider the diagnosis of PD.

There are no specific tests for PD. Brain imaging (MRI or CT) and blood tests are useful to eliminate other potential illnesses. These include: Normal Pressure Hydrocephalus, stroke, and other rare metabolic/genetic problems. In appropriate patients, blood may be drawn to screen for the "Parkin" gene through a commercial laboratory. Mutations in this gene usually result in young-onset PD, and the patient may have an affected sibling due to its autosomal recessive inheritance. Gene testing for Parkin might therefore be undertaken in a 45-year-old patient with parkinsonism and resting tremor, and an older sister diagnosed with PD in her forties. Other blood work in this setting may include a thyroid panel and a vitamin B12 level.

In the future, imaging tests that assess dopamine function in the brain may become more widely available. At this time, these tests (fluorodopa PET and β-CIT SPECT) are usually reserved for research applications.

When should I think about other types of parkinsonism?

Referrals early in the course of a parkinsonian type of illness are often made for a second opinion regarding diagnosis. At this time, patients and families may sense inconsistencies with the clinical diagnosis when compared to others with PD or descriptions found in literature. Often, further medical evaluation is necessary to eliminate other parkinsonism "masqueraders." Other causes of parkinsonism include Atypical Parkinsonism, drug-induced parkinsonism, and other heredodegenerative conditions. Drugs known to cause or worsen parkinsonism include anti-psychotics (neuroleptics), anti-emetics, and the antihypertensive agent, alpha-methyl-dopa. In addition, environmental toxins such as carbon monoxide, cyanide, carbon disulfide, manganese, lithium, and alcohol withdrawal have been associated with parkinsonian features.

Were there features on exam that lead to a diagnosis?

This patient has several features that are unusual for Parkinson's Disease. An important observation is that this man's tremor predated the onset of his walking and balance problem by almost eight years. Furthermore, the tremor sounds is an action tremor, and involved the voice, two common components of

Essential Tremor. With that symptom (tremor) explained, the diagnosis of PD becomes much less likely, although it is still important to see if the patient responds to anti-PD therapy – at adequate dosages. Although what is considered adequate is a matter of debate, a two-month trial of levodopa 300 – 400 mg/d. If no response, the dose can be escalated further and it is usually prudent not to conclude that there is no response until a dose as high as 1000 mg has been tried (if there are substantial symptoms).

How did you manage this patient's medication and what was the response?

Unfortunately, this man did not respond to levodopa and he then sought treatment options and evaluations from a number of other care providers. He has seen five neurologists in four different states who prescribed various PD medications without benefit. His gait disorder and balance difficulties did not respond to PD drugs, and progressed over time. In addition, he then developed difficulty with downgaze and is now thought to have Progressive Supranuclear Palsy. Thus in retrospect, this was an unusual case of an individual who had Essential Tremor, and later developed Progressive Supranuclear Palsy.

2) Initial Treatment:

Case Presentation: Hannah is a 42-year-old woman with a 12-month history of intermittent resting tremor of her right hand. The tremor tends to increase with anxiety or excitement, such as watching a sporting event, and if she concentrates, she can stop the tremor. She also has noticed a bothersome change in her handwriting, trouble buttoning, and some trouble tying her "wiggly" child's shoes. While she is able to complete all of the tasks required of her at home and at work, in the last several months she is aware that she is slowing down and is increasingly tired at the end of the day. On examination she has mild slowness in the right arm and leg, and walks with her right arm flexed at her side, but does not have difficulty with balance. There is mild rigidity on the right, and slight rigidity on the left.

Does she have to go on treatment?

Not necessarily. No medication has been proven to slow progression of PD and the exact best moment to introduce symptomatic medications in PD is not known. However, most experts agree that symptomatic medication should generally be introduced when the patient is having some functional disability. This woman's story is quite typical for the early PD patient. She has difficulty with handwriting and doing some tasks, so introduction of symptomatic therapy may be appropriate. In addition, it is possible that she is beginning to develop left sided symptoms (slight rigidity on the examination), and with bilateral symptoms, motor compensation becomes more difficult.

Is there a neuroprotective drug for Parkinson's disease?

No medication has been proven to slow the progression of PD. Selegiline has been shown to delay the need for levodopa, but this is likely due to its small symptomatic benefit. More recently, a "delayed-start" trial design with rasagiline found that patients who started the drug right away did better than those who waited six months. However, these data are still preliminary, and need to be confirmed in another trial. There are also several other medications that are currently being tested for potential neuroprotective effects including Coenzyme Q10 and creative.

Would progression of the disease be accelerated if there is delay in treatment?

There are no data to suggest delaying anti-parkinson medications would accelerate the progression of Parkinson's disease.

What medication should be introduced to improve this patient's symptoms?

Anticholinergic drugs such as trihexiphenidyl can improve tremor but provide little benefit for slowness and stiffness. Since this patient has symptoms beyond tremor, it is probably not the best choice for her. Medications that could be considered include MAO-B inhibitors, dopamine agonists, and levodopa. MAO-B inhibitors provide mild symptom benefit and have few side effects. Rasagiline appears to provide greater symptom benefit than selegiline. Dopamine agonists provide more symptom benefit than MAO-B inhibitors and are associated with less development of motor fluctuations and dyskinesias than levodopa, but have side effects that can include sleepiness, hallucinations, and edema.

In early disease, dopamine agonists provide almost as much symptomatic benefit as levodopa, but as the disease progresses levodopa is required to maintain control of symptoms. Dopamine agonists are commonly employed in early disease to control symptoms while delaying fluctuations and dyskinesia, especially in younger individuals. Levodopa provides good symptom benefit and is usually well tolerated. The disadvantage of levodopa is that its long-term use is associated with the development of motor fluctuations and dyskinesias. There is interest in whether the early introduction of a COMT inhibitor will reduce the incidence of motor fluctuations and dyskinesias. A clinical trial, STRIDE-PD, is currently underway to test this hypothesis.

3) Motor Fluctuations:

The early PD patient enjoys a robust and prolonged response to levodopa therapy, but within five years 30-80% of patients notice "wearing-off" or end-of-dose deterioration in mobility. The next phase of levodopa response occurs when peak levodopa levels produce involuntary movements or dyskinesias. Besides motor fluctuations, autonomic, sensory, and psychological symptoms sometimes fluctuate in response to levodopa fluctuations in the blood. "On" symptoms may include euphoria, sweating, hypotension, and nausea; "off" symptoms may include dysphoria, hypertension, difficulty initiating urination or defecation, excessive sweating, paresthesias, and pain.

Case Presentation: Agnes is a 76-year-old woman with PD for the last 13 years. Recently, she has noticed difficulty sleeping and wakes up frequently in the night with leg cramping. Her medication regimen consists of carbidopa/levodopa 25/100 at 8:00 am, noon, and 4:00 pm. She also admits that she will occasionally "sneak" a pill at 8:00 pm. Typically, she awakens with painful cramping at about 7:00 am each morning, and this continues until about 30 minutes after her 8:00 am levodopa pill. She feels well all morning, but will often have cramping return toward lunchtime. The cramping is usually gone by early afternoon, but will return before her 4:00 pm medication, and will become increasingly worse as the evening progresses. She does not report any involuntary movements. (Figure 1)

Dosing Diary Response Curve

7	8	9	10	11	12	1	2	3	4	5	6
		on	on	on		on	on	on		on	on
	off				off				off		

Medication Schedule

	25/100				25/100				25/100		

Figure 1. *ON = moving normally; off = Parkinson's symptoms limiting mobility; 25/100 = carbidopa/levodopa 25/100*

What treatment options are available?

This patient demonstrates a typical "wearing-off" dystonia, in this example a side effect of low levels of levodopa. The "dosing diary" demonstrates cramping at the end of the levodopa dosing cycle. Although in this case, the patient primary "off" symptom is cramping, the same considerations would apply for other "off" symptoms including decreased mobility.

Increasing the levodopa dose of 25/100 to 1½ tablets at 8:00 am, noon and 4:00 pm and adding a tablet at 8:00 pm, or by switching to levodopa/carbidopa/entacapone 100/25/200 at these dosing times may treat the daytime problems. Another approach could be giving the medication more often (carbidopa/levodopa 25/100 at 7:00 am, 10:00 am, 1:00 pm , 4:00 pm and 7:00 pm), or the patient could be placed on carbidopa/levodopa CR 50/200 tablets, one at 7:00 am, noon, and 5:00 pm. Another option is the addition of a dopamine agonist. Once an initial change is made, its effects will have to be assessed and further changes may be required.

Dosing Diary Response Curve

7	8	9	10	11	12	1	2	3	4	5	6
			dys				dys				dys
	on	on		on	on	on		on	on	on	
off											

Medication Schedule

7	8	9	10	11	12	1	2	3	4	5	6
	1½ 25/100				1½ 25/100				1½ 25/100		

Figure 2. *Dys = dyskinesia; ON = moving normally; off = Parkinson's symptoms limiting mobility; 25/100 = carbidopa/levodopa 25/100*

In this case, carbidopa/levodopa was increased to 1½ tablets of 25/100 at 8,12,4 and 1 tablet at 8 pm. She returns in one month and reports less leg cramping during the day, but continued sleep difficulty and cramping at night. In addition, she now has involuntary movements (dyskinesia) of her head at 10:00 am, 2:00 pm, and 6:00 pm every day. (Figure 2)

On this regimen the patient exhibits simple motor fluctuations and dyskinesias that are easily correlated to levodopa dosing. At this time point there are several options that might help smooth her clinical response. These include: give smaller doses of 25/100 carbidopa/levodopa more frequently (every three hours), switch to levodopa/carbidopa/entacapone100/25/200 (every four hours), or return to the previous levodopa dosing schedule and add another medication. (Figure 3) Since one and half tablets of carbidopa/levodopa 25/100 produced dyskinesia and one tablet does not last a full four hours, a reasonable option would be to give one tablet every three hrs or to add entacapone 200 mg to one tablet of carbidopa/levodopa given every three and half to four hrs. This would potentially eliminate "peak dose" dyskinesia and "wearing-off" problems. Trying a levodopa/carbidopa CR regimen may be less ideal because variability in absorption may make it hard to control both fluctuations and dyskinesia. Another alternative would be to return to the original carbidopa/levodopa 25/100 regimen, and add another medication. This could be a dopamine agonist, an MAO-B inhibitor, or amantadine.

Dosing Diary Response Curve

7	8	9	10	11	12	1	2	3	4	5	6
on	on	on	on	on	on	on	on	on	on	on	on

Medication Schedule

7	8	9	10	11	12	1	2	3	4	5	6
25/100			25/100			25/100			25/100		
ENT 25/100				ENT 25/100				ENT 25/100			
DA 25/100				DA 25/100				DA 25/100			

Figure 3. *ON = moving normally; 25/100 = carbidopa/levodopa 25/100; ENT = entacapone 200 mg, DA = dopamine agonist. The figure illustrates the 3 different dosing strategies discussed above.*

How should I take my medicine in relation to my meals?

There are two basic factors to consider when taking medications for Parkinson's disease. The most frequently mentioned problem concerns dietary interaction of protein and levodopa. This condition affects less than 20% of patients, and significantly affects less than 5% of patients taking levodopa. Levodopa is an amino acid. A string of amino acids that are chemically connected make up a protein. Thus, if levodopa is ingested with a meal of high protein, the protein will be converted into amino acids, and through competition for absorption from the gut to the bloodstream, the effective dosage of levodopa is reduced.

Clinically, a Parkinson patient may notice a lack of boost from carbidopa/levodopa when taken with food, and when severe, may notice a decline in mobility after eating a high protein meal. If this is a concern, taking carbidopa/levodopa on an empty stomach, 30 minutes before or 60 minutes after eating is suggested. If a severe problem, nutritional counseling is an excellent way to balance protein ingestion with levodopa intake, and may offer further help.

The most common problem with meals and medication is the size of the meals. Parkinson's disease slows the motility of the gastro-intestinal tract, and if medications are taken with a large meal, absorption may be delayed, regardless of protein concentration or type of medication.

I seem to have more pain and muscle cramping than I used to, especially in the mornings. Is pain a common part of PD?

Pain affects up to half of all patients with Parkinson's disease. It may occur during "off" periods, when medication is not working and PD symptoms return, or during "on" periods, when it is working.

Off-period pain is most often due to rigidity (muscle stiffness) or dystonia. Limbs that are not moved through their full range of motion may become painful. This is especially common in the morning, since the effects of anti-PD medications usually wear off over night, and you may spend the last few hours of sleep in the off state. Painful foot cramping (dystonia), especially in the morning, is very common in PD patients. This is often helped by the addition of a dopamine agonist, as a bedtime dose may last until morning.
Some PD patients also have restless legs syndrome, which causes painful or uncomfortable feelings in the legs, especially at night, that are improved with movement of the legs. Dopamine agonists are also helpful to relieve restless legs syndrome.

Pain may also occur during "on" periods. Dyskinesias, or uncontrolled movements, may become painful or uncomfortable if they are severe enough or are associated with dystonia. Other kinds of pain in PD may include gastrointestinal pain, neck pain, headache, and a general feeling of pain or unease throughout the body.

What can I do to reduce my pain?

Identifying the cause and timing of the pain is an important first step. Off-period pain, including early morning pain or foot dystonia, is usually caused by low levels of levodopa or other dopaminergic medications. Using a dopamine agonist or possibly a sustained-release formulation of levodopa may help, as can taking a dose of drug an hour before rising in the morning. A single injection of apomorphine just before rising is another option, since this drug works much quicker than other dopamine agonists, but is usually reserved for more difficult cases. For on-period pain, adjusting medications may offer some relief. Pain caused by dyskinesias or dystonia may be lessened by amantadine, which reduces dyskinesias.

As with muscle and joint pain from other causes, massage and application of heat to the affected area may reduce pain. Physical therapy and moderate exercise may help as well. Over-the-counter pain medications can also be tried.

My husband has been falling a lot lately, to the point where I'm afraid every time he goes out. Can this be improved by medications or other treatments?

Falling is an unfortunately common occurrence in advanced Parkinson's disease. It is the result of a complex mix of factors, only some of which can be satisfactorily treated. Impaired balance, slowed movements, stiffness, and slow switching of attention when balance is threatened all contribute to the risk for falling. Studies show that levodopa can help prevent falls to some extent, principally by increasing speed of movement and reducing stiffness. However, impaired balance per se usually does not improve with medication changes.

Medications that cause confusion may increase the risk for falling. If you are experiencing falls, it is important to have your physician examine and adjust your medications with this in mind. Regular exercise is valuable in and of itself, and can help improve reflexes and strength. This can help reduce falls as well. A physical therapist familiar with the challenges of PD can help design an exercise program. An occupational therapist may be able to suggest modifications in the home or work environment to reduce the risk of injury from falls. Vitamin D to strengthen bones may reduce the risk of fracture. Be sure to consult your physician about all of these options.

Is freezing a symptom of "off" time? Are there any treatments that can help this?

Episodic freezing occurs in up to half of advanced PD patients. The person may freeze when trying to start from a standstill, when turning, while passing through a narrow opening such as a doorway, or upon reaching his destination. It may occur during "off" time or "on" time. When the problem occurs during "off" time, it is likely to improve with medication changes that reduce "off" time. When freezing occurs during "on" time, it may be difficult to improve. It may be helpful to work with an occupational therapist who can examine the specific situations in which freezing is most likely. For some patients, rearranging the furniture to avoid tight spaces may help, while for others laying out step-length markers on the floor is beneficial. These kinds of strategies may help the patient reduce the likelihood of freezing.

4) Treatment of Dyskinesias:

Ray is a 74-year-old man with a nine-year history of Parkinson's disease, initially treated with a dopamine agonist, who has had motor fluctuations, dyskinesias, and painful early-morning leg cramping for three years. The patient had been reasonably well controlled for the three years prior to evaluation. His medications include carbidopa/levodopa 25/100 tid, entacapone 200 mg tid, pergolide 1.25 mg tid, selegiline 5 mg qd, and zolpidem 10 mg qhs.

During an office evaluation in October 2003, he was found to have agitation, anxiety, and tremulousness. In addition, during a prolonged evaluation he exhibited both wearing-off with dystonic posturing of his right arm and leg, and peak-dose dyskinesia dosing which he "felt like he was coming out of his skin."

Because of concerns regarding cardiac valve damage, the patient was switched from pergolide 1.25 mg tid to pramipexole 1 mg tid over a three-week period. During this time he noted no change in his mobility, dyskinesias, or off-periods. Unfortunately, he did notice significant alopecia. Because of this he was changed from pramipexole 1 mg tid to ropinirole 6 mg tid. The hair loss stabilized, and his motor symptoms remained unchanged. At this time, amantadine 100 mg bid was added to his medical regimen in an effort to smooth his response and improve both wearing-off and dyskinesia. He then reported increased mobility with less troublesome dyskinesia, and less painful off-periods. Nonetheless, early morning foot dystonia continued to be his most frustrating PD symptom.

In September 2004, because of his increasing difficulty with painful delay to on in the morning and unpredictable off periods, he was initiated on subcutaneous apomorphine injections. He was titrated to a 4 mg dosage and he self-administered this each morning upon awakening and as needed when he turned off through the day. The early morning apomorphine injection was very helpful in reducing his morning dystonia.

List of Medications (including dosage and interval)

Carbidopa/levodopa 25/100,
2 tablets at 7am and 1 tablet at 10am, 1pm, 4pm, 7pm, and 10pm

Carbidopa/levodopa CR 50/200,
1/2 tablet at 7am, 10am, 1pm, 4pm, 7pm, and 10pm

Ropinirole 6 mg tid
Selegiline 5 mg every morning
Amantadine 100 mg at 7am and 1pm
Apomorphine 4 mg sc q am, and prn

Diagnosis

Advanced Parkinson's disease with:

1) motor fluctuations including unpredictable wearing-off
2) troublesome peak-dose dyskinesias, and
3) painful early morning foot dystonia (associated with delayed time to on),

Questions:

What causes dyskinesia?

Dyskinesias are a combination of disease duration and levodopa exposure. Dopamine agonists alone rarely cause wearing-off or dyskinesia.

Can dyskinesias be prevented?

Using dopamine agonists as initial dopamine therapy and delaying the introduction of levodopa can delay dyskinesias, but eventually most patients will need levodopa to maintain best mobility. Most patients treated with levodopa for more than five years will have some dyskinesia.

What treatments are used for dyskinesias?

Amantadine can reduce dyskinesia. In addition, reduction of dopaminergic medications will result in less dyskinesia but may result in more "off" time or worsening of PD symptoms.

5) Medication Induced Hallucinations in Parkinson's Disease:

JR is a 67-year-old man with an eight-year history of PD treated with a combination of pramipexole and carbidopa/levodopa. He is accompanied to the office by his family, who report a recent history of increasing visual hallucinations and paranoia. His hallucinations were most common in the evening and consisted of seeing people who would talk to him. Initially, he recognized that the hallucinations were not real but recently he has been acting on them. In addition to his hallucinations, the patient has developed paranoia and is suspecting his wife of infidelity.

The patient has been on his current medication schedule for the past six months. He has a past history of vivid dreams and nightmares. Over the past year he has become more forgetful and during the past month he has developed hallucinations and paranoia. Attempts to lower his medications improved his hallucinations but resulted in a significant worsening of his motor function.

The patient was placed on a single bedtime dose of quetiapine and this was escalated as tolerated to a dose of 100 mg. With this he had improvement of his sleep and resolution of his hallucinations and paranoia.

How do you treat hallucinations and paranoia?

Symptoms of psychosis pose major concerns for family members and caregivers of PD patients. With increasing cognitive symptoms or nightmares, simplification of anti-PD therapy should be considered. Elimination of amantadine, dopamine agonists, and anticholinergic drugs may be helpful. In many instances simplification of medications to carbidopa/levodopa alone, will allow for continued mobility with less hallucinations. Quetiapine is often very helpful in reducing or eliminating hallucinations, and if necessary, clozapine can be used although it requires blood count monitoring.

6) Sleep Disorders:

Insomnia in PD may result from difficulty with sleep initiation or with sleep maintenance, and may be worsened by motor limitations or tremor. Difficulty with sleep initiation may be improved with hypnotics, tricyclic antidepressants, benzodiazepines, diphenhydramine, or chloral hydrate. However, if the patient reports limb cramping, particularly in the "parkinsonian" side, this sleep difficulty may be a result of "wearing-off" from levodopa, and a bedtime dose of carbidopa/levodopa CR may be helpful. Nocturnal urinary frequency sometimes responds to a synthetic anti-diuretic hormone (DDAVP 2 mg) at bedtime. Nightmares often improve with clonazepam 0.5 - 1.0 mg at bedtime.

Agnes (Case 2) is now happy with her improved motor ability during the day, but now strongly desires to address her sleep problems and early morning foot cramping. In this instance the addition of amitriptyline 10-25 mg at bedtime may help both the sleep and foot-cramping problem, and would be a reasonable choice. If, however the patient has memory difficulties or problems with urinary retention this drug should be avoided. Treatment with a dopamine agonist or baclofen 20 mg at bedtime and in the early morning may alleviate symptoms of foot cramping. Clonazepam 0.5 - 1.0 mg may be useful in treating sleep problems in some patients.

What is REM behavior disorder?

This is a common problem in PD patients, and often associated with nightmares, screaming and fighting during sleep. This condition is often frightening to a bed partner, and may be associated with sleep disruption to all. Treatment is usually with clonazepam.

Case presentation: KH is a 62-year-old retired pilot with a seven-year history of PD. He initially did extremely well on levodopa only (a drug approved by the FAA for licensed pilots), but with increasing motor fluctuations and some mild dyskinesias, sought disability as a commercial pilot. During the first year after retiring, pramipexole was added to his levodopa regimen and his motor fluctuations, dyskinesias, and general mobility markedly improved. However, with time he continued to increase his levodopa and pramipexole to maintain his active lifestyle. One day he was involved in a motor vehicle accident.

Mr. H lives in a gated community, in which his home is approximately 200 meters from an entry gate. One afternoon he was preparing to go for a round of golf, and after hanging up the phone, and placing his golf clubs in the trunk, he immediately set off for his destination. He reports he got in his car, drove out his driveway, and apparently fell asleep, without warning, and ran into the automatic gate control. While he remembers lowering the automatic garage door, be does not completely recall backing out of the driveway or moving toward his community exit. He estimates the time it would take for him to drive this distance would be less than five seconds.

This experience is consistent with a "sleep attack", or sudden onset sleep that can occur during treatment with a dopamine agonist, and to a lesser extent with levodopa. While treatment is usually withdrawal of the dopamine agonist, this patient did not tolerate stopping pramipexole. He admitted that he was actually taking 5-6 mg of pramipexole per day and found that by reducing his dose to 3 mg per day he experienced no further episodes.

What are sleep attacks?

This uncommon condition is described as a sudden, irresistible urge to sleep, and is most often associated with dopamine agonists, usually within the first several months after dosage increase beyond an initial therapeutic dosage (e.g. pramipexole 3 mg/daily). Reduction or elimination of the offending agent may resolve the problem. In some patients treatment with modafinil is helpful.

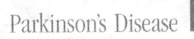

CHAPTER 13

QUESTIONS FREQUENTLY ASKED BY PATIENTS

Theresa A. Zesiewicz and Robert A. Hauser

Is exercise important for patients with Parkinson's disease?

Exercise is extremely important in Parkinson's disease. Exercise helps maintain the best possible function in the face of a progressive disorder. The saying, "Use it or lose it" applies. For example, a walking regimen helps maintain the ability to walk. In addition, exercise provides the added benefits of improving mood, energy level, and sleep.

Have studies demonstrated that exercise is beneficial?

Yes, exercise programs have been shown to produce improvement in gait, grip strength, and motor coordination [1]. In one study, a 13-week exercise program consisting of supervised and unsupervised home exercises was associated with significant improvement in gait [2]. Another study demonstrated improvement in range of motion as a result of an exercise program consisting of climbing stairs, hitting a punching bag, and catching a ball [3].

What types of exercises are important?

Exercises for mobility, stretching, and strengthening are all important. Mobility exercises help maintain walking ability. A stretching regimen improves flexibility and helps fight the tendency for stooped posture. Increased strength will help maintain mobility and function even as slowness and stiffness progress.

How often should I exercise?

At least three or four times per week and preferably every day. The amount of time spent exercising each day is partly a function of tolerance, but most patients should exercise for at least twenty minutes per session.

If you cannot tolerate twenty minutes at a time, divide it up through the day, and try to build up your tolerance. Patients with early disease can usually tolerate 40 minutes to an hour of exercise per session.

Doesn't the exercise regimen depend on the stage of the disease?

Yes, the type of exercise that's right for a particular person depends on functional ability. A young person with early disease may play tennis, swim laps, jog, or ride a bicycle. For patients who are a little older or who have a little more advanced disease, exercise activities might include golf, light swimming, walking in a pool, or using a stationary bicycle or rowing machine. For patients with moderate disease, a walking regimen is very important. During hot or cold weather, many patients like to walk indoors. A shopping mall is often a good place to walk because it is temperature-controlled and the floor is usually flat and not slippery. Walkers can be used in a mall if necessary. For patients who are unable to walk, mobility, stretching and strengthening exercises that can be done in a chair are appropriate.

It is important to find physical activities that you like to do so that you will continue them over time. A long-term program is necessary because studies have shown that the benefit of exercise is lost when patients discontinue their regimen [4]. Engage in physical activity that is at the right level for you. Activities that create undue risk should be avoided. The importance of moderate exercise cannot be stressed enough and it is not believed that overdoing it, such as training for a marathon, is either necessary or helpful.

Are rehabilitation programs helpful?

Rehabilitation programs can help tailor a regimen to suit your needs. A physical therapist will evaluate your function, abilities, and limitations and will design a program based on that evaluation. In addition, rehabilitation programs give you a "jump start", to get you going on your exercise program. However, you must keep up the program once you have completed rehabilitation to maintain the benefit. Be sure to receive clear instructions as to what regimen is recommended once you have completed the initial program.

If you are considering a rehabilitation program, it is recommended that you meet with the personnel to discuss what services will be provided. You will also want to know the cost, and what may be covered by insurance.

What types of therapists make up a rehabilitation program?

Physical therapists perform a functional evaluation, design a physical rehabilitation program, and assist you in carrying out the program. They might also recommend assistive devices for ambulating such as a walker. Occupational therapists perform a functional evaluation concentrating on fine finger and hand movements. They recommend exercises and adaptive devices to improve hand and arm function.

Occupational therapists also perform home evaluations to determine if modifications would be helpful. They might determine that handrails are needed in the shower to help prevent falls or that a trapeze device would help you to get out of bed or turn over at night.

Speech therapists evaluate voice amplitude and clarity. They often provide speech exercises and teach patients techniques to help them communicate better. Speech therapists also evaluate swallowing. Swallowing is assessed by observation and in some cases a special test called a barium swallow will be needed. Based on the swallowing evaluation, a speech therapist will make recommendations regarding optimal food texture and thickening liquids, and teach techniques to make swallowing easier and safer.

I have Parkinson's disease and am having trouble with balance. My physician recommends that I get a walking device. Which one should I purchase?

Wheeled walkers may prevent falls in patients with balance difficulty and can improve mobility [5]. Two, three, and four-wheeled walkers are available. The 3-wheeled walker is shaped like a triangle. One study compared 2- and 3-wheeled walkers and found the 3-legged, 3-wheeled models preferable. Subjects walked faster and had greater maneuverability with the 3-wheeled walker [5]. We prefer the 3-legged, 3-wheeled walker with hand brakes for patients who are able to use it. Before purchasing a walking device, visit a medical supply store and try out different varieties. Determine which one works best for you.

I have Parkinson's disease and I am speaking too softly. What can I do to improve this?

Approximately 60 to 90% of PD patients exhibit speech or voice abnormalities [6] including reduced volume, diminished articulation, decreased variation in tone, tremor [7], or hoarseness [8]. Patients may lose clarity of speech and articulation of consonants is less precise. Particularly difficult are the sounds of the letters k,g,f,v,s, and z [9]. Just as there may be decreased dexterity in fine finger movements, there is also a loss of dexterity in the muscles involved in articulation. Decreased control and strength of airflow, and rigidity of the laryngeal muscles may also contribute to speech difficulty [8].

In some patients there is bowing of the vocal cords so that they do not lie in contact with each other to capture airflow and vibrate. For these patients, collagen injections into the vocal cords may remarkably improve speech [10]. ENT specialists perform this procedure as well as a specialized evaluation to assess whether the procedure might offer benefit. Increasing antiparkinsonian mediation may improve speech but there are often limitations as to how much benefit can be achieved with medication adjustments alone [11]. Voice rehabilitation is beneficial in improving vocal intensity and articulation [12]. Ask your physician to refer you to a speech therapist for exercises you can perform at home.

How can I maximize the benefit of my visit to the doctor?

Recognize that the time the doctor can spend with you is limited. The better prepared you are, the better able your doctor will be to address your questions and concerns. Bring a list of all your medications, the doses, and the times you take them. It may be helpful to bring your medications in their labelled containers in case questions arise.

You should tell the doctor what aspect of your Parkinson's disease is currently causing you the most difficulty. You may also want to discuss the next one or two biggest problems. We suggest that you determine in advance what three problems you most want to discuss. It is usually not possible to address more than three problems at a single visit. You might mention more than three if they are important to you, but focus on three or less to be addressed and discussed.

If something is on your mind, particularly medication changes that you think might be beneficial, be sure to bring it up for consideration. If the doctor suggests changes that you do not think will be helpful, be sure to tell him so that he will have a chance to discuss it further or reconsider his recommendations.

I have motor fluctuations and dyskinesia. What additional information will my doctor want?

If you are experiencing motor fluctuations, your doctor will want to know how long it takes for your levodopa to start to work, and how long the benefit lasts. He will want to know how much of the day, while you are awake, the medication is providing benefit (ON time) and how much of the day you are not experiencing benefit because the medication has worn off (OFF time). If you are having dyskinesia (twisting, turning movements) he will want to know how much of the day they are present, and how troublesome they are, if at all. He will also want to know what causes you more difficulty, OFF time or dyskinesia.

I don't like anyone else in the room with me during my doctor's visit. Is that OK?

We strongly believe that someone else should be in the room with you during your office visit, preferably a spouse or caregiver. It is often valuable for the doctor to get additional information from a second person who knows how you are doing at home. Another perspective may help emphasize certain problems. In addition, your spouse or caregiver may have their own questions or concerns that need to be addressed. It is also helpful to have two people listen to the discussion in case one forgets what was said after the visit is over.

What should I take with me when I leave the doctor's office?

You should receive written instructions detailing any medication changes and these should be clear to you before you leave the office. If the instructions are not clear, ask for additional clarification. You may want to refer to the written instructions at home in case you can not remember or if uncertainty arises later. A copy of your written instructions should be placed in your medical chart so that this is available if you call with questions or a problem occurs.

How often should I see my doctor for my Parkinson's disease?

Patients who are stable and doing reasonably well might be seen about every four months. This usually provides the opportunity to make medication changes before there has been too much progression in symptoms. Most patients should be seen no less frequently than every six months. If visits are less often than six months, disease progression without medication adjustment may cause unnecessary discomfort and disability. Patients are commonly seen more frequently than every four months if multiple medication adjustments are required so as not to waste time. If a new medication is introduced that needs to be monitored, or if further adjustments are expected, the next visit is scheduled sooner.

My doctor gave me a prescription for a new medication. I bought one month supply only to find I could not tolerate the medication. How can I avoid this happening in the future?

When a new medication is prescribed, ask your doctor if samples are available to see if you can tolerate it before buying it. You can also ask your pharmacist to initially dispense a few days supply before filling the rest of the prescription.

My medication is very expensive and my insurance plan does not cover it. Can I get help with the cost of my medication?

If the cost of medication is an issue, be sure to let your doctor know. He can then consider cost more strongly when he formulates a treatment plan. Some medications are more expensive than others. Ask your doctor about generic medications. In most cases, if a generic formulation is available it will be less expensive than the name brand. Remember that a generic does not always contain exactly the same amount of medication as the name brand even if the pill is the same "dose". Patients who are sensitive to small changes in dose may prefer the name brand.

Most pharmaceutical companies have programs to provide medication for patients that are truly unable to afford it. An application that includes your financial information can be submitted to the company to see if you qualify for the program. Ask your physician for the name, address, and phone number of the company that distributes the medication, and contact the company.

My physician has diagnosed me with Parkinson's disease, but I would like a second opinion. Where should I go to get one?

Contact one of the information and referral sources listed at the end of this chapter. They will provide the name of a Movement Disorder or Parkinson's disease specialist, who will be happy to provide a second opinion. Do not be afraid or embarrassed to obtain a second opinion, and bring all scans and records with you.

Should I join a support group?

Support groups are very valuable. They are a tremendous source of information regarding the disease, coping mechanisms, treatment options, local doctors, and support services. They provide a sense of community and shared experience. Support groups serve as a forum to express frustrations and to share your knowledge.

Support groups are most helpful if they include others like you. Some supports group are specifically for young or newly diagnosed patients.

I am scheduled to undergo surgery for another medical problem. Is there anything special I need to know?

Because of possible serious complications due to the interaction of MAO-B inhibitors (selegiline and rasagiline) and anesthesia or narcotics, these medications should be discontinued at least ten days prior to elective surgery. You should discuss with your doctors how you should handle your other antiparkinsonian medications. In order to avoid worsening mobility, breathing, and swallowing that may occur if patients are off medications for more than a few hours, antiparkinsonian medications should usually be taken right up to the time of surgery and reinstituted as soon after surgery as possible. Immediately after surgery your stomach and intestine may not be functioning and absorbing medications normally, and you may find that even though you are taking your medications you may not get a response.

While in the hospital, patients with confusion or hallucinations may experience a worsening of these symptoms due to the unfamiliar environment. Pain medications, sedatives, and infections can also worsen confusion and hallucinations. Because of these potential problems, it is recommended that patients with advanced PD have their surgery at a hospital where a neurologist who is familiar with them and knowledgeable about PD is available to provide care.

Am I at increased risk for complications from surgery because of my disease?

Patients with more advanced disease have a higher complication rate following surgery. One study found that the average length of hospital stay was more than two days longer for Parkinson's disease patients than non-parkinsonian patients[13]. Parkinson's disease patients had more urinary tract infections, pneumonia, and other bacterial infections. This higher complication rate probably reflects diminished mobility, breathing, and swallowing[14]. Patients who are immobile may have urinary catheters in place longer, thereby causing urinary tract infections[13]. It is important to have catheters and other lines taken out as soon as they are no longer needed and to be out of bed as soon and as often as is feasible. In considering whether you should have a particular operation, you and your doctor should weigh the relative benefits and risks in light of this higher complication rate.

My husband has Parkinson's disease and I am concerned about his driving. What should I do?

Driving requires high level motor and thinking skills, good judgment, and quick reaction times. Advanced PD and cognitive impairment are associated with higher accident rates[15]. Unfortunately, the patient is often unaware of diminished driving ability and it usually falls on the spouse or other family members to detect driving problems. This can cause conflict within a family, as some patients are unwilling to stop driving even when told it is unsafe. A driving simulator test can provide an objective assessment of driving ability, or the patient can be referred to a motor vehicle agency for a driving evaluation. If you have concerns about your spouse's driving ability, let your physician know. Although sympathetic to the loss of independence that comes with loss of driving ability, patient safety and the safety of everyone on the road is the paramount consideration.

I am 57-years-old and I am having difficulty doing my job. I have just been diagnosed with Parkinson's disease. Should I continue working or should I consider disability or early retirement ?

Avoid a hasty decision. Treatment may improve your symptoms such that you may be able to do your job without much difficulty. It is usually wise to gauge your response to medication before making any long-term employment decisions.

If you feel your job is threatened because of poor performance, it is important to convey this to your doctor.

Approximately thirty to forty percent of PD patients stop working early[16,17]. However, lost wages and earnings are a potential family burden and source of stress[18]. You will want to carefully weigh the pros and cons of retiring early. An important consideration is medical insurance. Unless special arrangements are made, you will probably lose the medical insurance that came with your job if you discontinue your employment. In the US, If you are under age for medicare it may be extremely expensive or impossible to purchase new medical insurance.

Can I get social security disability?

Social security disability is for individuals who are permanently and completely disabled, and unable to engage in any gainful employment. Because the criteria are so strict, the process often takes a long time and many patients with Parkinson's disease are denied disability benefits the first time they apply. The key is to be persistent and reapply if you meet eligibility criteria. An attorney who specializes in social security disability can help.

I developed Parkinson's disease five years ago. I'm worried about the emotional impact the disease might have on my spouse.

Studies have demonstrated that the amount and type of stress experienced by a caregiver progresses and changes with each stage of the disease[19]. Caregiver stress is relatively low when the patient is in the first two stages of disease, although worry begins to emerge in stage II. When the patient is in stage III, caregivers experience increased tension and frustration, often stemming from communication problems and role conflict.

In stages IV and V, caregivers experience increased stress due to economic burdens, lack of resources, and feelings of manipulation. These stressors are very real and can have a profound impact on the patient, the caregiver, and their relationship.

Support groups, respite care, educational resources, and professional services may help to reduce strain on family members of PD patients. A social worker or psychologist may be of benefit to provide support and counselling. If possible, it is usually helpful for the caregiver to maintain independent activities and friends. Scheduled breaks from caregiving are also valuable. Expectations placed on the caregiver must be realistic and not overwhelming. Although many caregivers attempt to put forth superhuman efforts, this may cause more problems than it solves. It is often better to obtain additional help as offered in an assisted care living facility or nursing home.

Should I take vitamins?

No vitamin is known to provide benefit for Parkinson's disease. Although there is interest as to whether vitamin E might slow the progression of PD, studies to date have not provided evidence that it does so [20]. We usually suggest that PD patients take a single multivitamin each day as we recommend for everyone.

What foods should I eat now that I've been diagnosed with Parkinson's disease?

Dietary protein interferes with the absorption of levodopa from the gut and its transport into the brain [21]. However, only patients with advanced disease who are very sensitive to small changes in levodopa absorption need to be concerned about this. Most patients should simply concentrate on eating a healthy diet. Increased fiber, fruits, and vegetables help prevent constipation. There is a tendency for patients to lose weight over time, so individuals of normal weight should strive to maintain it. Obese individuals will want to prudently lose weight so that mobility can be maintained as the disease progresses. Overly aggressive or quick weight loss should be avoided. Special low protein, protein redistributed, or balanced protein diets may help patients with advanced disease who find that they lose medication benefit when they eat a meal that includes protein. It is still important to take in enough protein to maintain overall health. We recommend consultation with a dietitian for patients who might benefit from a protein-modified diet.

How are new medications developed?

Research is what creates new and better treatments. Research that involves chemicals and cells in laboratories is called basic research and research that involves people is called clinical research. Promising new medications are initially discovered and developed in research laboratories. The medication is then tested in animals. If the medication is demonstrated to be safe and effective in animals, it may be tested in people.

In the initial phase of clinical research, the medication is evaluated in normal individuals who volunteer to be part of the testing program. If the medication is demonstrated to be safe in normal volunteers, it may then be tested in patients. In sophisticated clinical trials, patients consent to receive pills that could be the real medication being tested or a fake (placebo) that contains no active medication. The reason this is done is because patients improve when they receive a placebo. This is called the placebo effect.

In part, the placebo effect is due to psychological factors and in part due to the way patients are evaluated. Because of this, if only the real medication were given, doctors could not tell if improvement was really an effect of the medication or due to the placebo effect. We therefore compare the improvement in patients who received the real medication to the improvement in patients who received placebo. If the real medication provided more improvement than the placebo, we know it is the difference in improvement that is due to the medication because everything else was handled in exactly the same way. If both groups improve the same amount then the medication did not provide any benefit.

I do not want to take a placebo.

Clinical studies that include a placebo are designed to minimize patient discomfort and risk. Some studies are for patients with very early disease, before treatment is required. In these studies, patients have the luxury of being able to take a placebo because there is minimal disability and other medications are not needed. Other studies are designed for patients who are on antiparkinsonian medications and need them to maintain benefit. In these clinical trials the placebo (or medication under study) is added to the medications the patient is already taking.

Most clinical trials are designed for patients who are doing reasonably well or for those patients who are not doing well but for whom additional benefit cannot be achieved with currently available treatments. Although many patients improve in clinical trials you cannot count on getting better. If you are in need of more medication and would be unhappy if you stayed the same through the trial, you should not enter the study until your medications have been adjusted and you are doing better. Of course, there are many different study designs, and if your other antiparkinsonian medications can be increased during the trial, there may be even less concern regarding a placebo. Discuss the details of the study with your doctor.

Should I participate in a clinical trial?

This is a very individual decision. However, the value of clinical trials cannot be underestimated. Clinical trials allow new medications and procedures to be tested and hopefully approved for patient use. We are able to use the medications we have now because other patients participated in the clinical trials needed to assess these medications. You may participate in a trial of a medication that will help you and others later on. This is one way to play an active role in fighting the disease. We also find that we get to know our patients who participate in clinical trials very well because we see them frequently. There is usually no charge for the care you receive in a clinical trial.

Are there reasons not to participate in clinical trials?

Some clinical trials are easier than others. They differ in their duration, frequency of visits, and how long each evaluation takes. Some may be too demanding for you. In addition, all medications have potential side effects and it is possible to experience a side effect in a clinical trial. There is usually a mechanism built into the study to deal with this possibility. The medication might be discontinued or the dose lowered. In some cases the side effect is treated with another medication. The further along a drug is in its clinical testing the more that is known about it. Conversely, there may be less known about a medication when it is first tested in patients. Ask your doctor to put these issues in perspective for you for the particular study you are considering.

I am interested in participating in a clinical trial. How do I do this?

Expert Movement Disorder Centers generally conduct the most clinical Parkinson's disease research. The information resource centers at the end of this chapter can refer you to an Expert Center and may also have information about national and local clinical trials. You may also want to call your local university medical school for the names and phone numbers of Movement Disorders experts in your area.

I am interested in donating money to research on Parkinson's disease.

Movement Disorder Centers and national organizations are delighted to accept donations to support research.

What else?

It is very important to keep a positive mental outlook. Do your part to eat right, exercise, and get enough sleep. Find a good doctor who knows a lot about Parkinson's disease and whom you like and trust. Do what you can to support research. Tremendous advances have been made in the recent past and the future looks extremely bright. An understanding of what causes the disease is close at hand. Understanding the cause will lead to a cure.

Chapter 13 - FAQ REFERENCES

1. Palmer S, Mortimer JA, Webster DD et al. Exercise therapy for Parkinson's disease. Arc Phys Med Rehabil 1986;67:741-745.

2. Szkely BC, Kosanovich NN, Sheppard W. Adjunctive treatment in Parkinson's disease: physical therapy and comprehensive group therap. Rehabil Lit 1982;43:72-76

3. Bilovit DS. Establishing physical objectives in rehabilitation of patients with Parkinson's disease (gymnastic activities). Phys The Rev 1956;36:176-178.

4. Comella CL, Stebbins GT, Brown-Toms N, Goetz CG. Physical Therapy and Parkinson's disease: a controlled clinical trial. Neurology 1994;44:376-378.

5. Mahoney J, Euhardy R, Carnes M. A comparison of a two-wheeled and three- wheeled walker in a geriatric population. JAGS 10992;40:735-736.

6. Logemann JA, Fisher HB, Boshes B et al. Frequency and co-occurrence of vocal tract dysfunctions in the speech of a large sample of Parkinson's patients. J Speech Hear Disord 1978;43:47-57.

7. Perez KS, Ramig LA, Smith ME et al. The Parkinson's larynx: tremor and videostroboscopic findings. J Voice 1996;10:354-361.

8. Hanson DG, Gerratt BR, Ward PH. Cinegraphic observations of laryngeal function in Parkinson's disease. Laryngoscope 1984;95:348-353.

9. Robbins JA, Logemann JA, Kishner HS. Swallowing and speech production in Parkinson's disease. Ann Neurol 1986;19:283-287.

10. Berke GS, Gerratt B, Kreiman J et al. Treatment of Parkison's hypophonia with percutaneous collagen augmentation. Laryncoscope 1999;108:1295-1299..

11. Jiang J, Lin E, Wang J et al. Glottographic measures before and after levadopa treatment in Parkinson's disease. Laryngoscope 1999;109:1287-1294.

12. DeAngelis EC, Mourao LF, Ferraz HB et al. Effect of voice rehabilitation on oral communication of Parkinson's disease. Acta Neurol Scand 1997;96:199-205.

13. Pepper PV, Goldstein MK. Postoperative complications in Parkinson's disease. JAGS 1999;47:967-972.

14. MacIntosh D. Respiratory dysfunction in Parkinson's disease. Prim Care 1977;4:441-445.

15. Dubinsky RM, Gray C. Husted D et al. Driving in Parkinson's disease. Neurology 1991;41:517-520.

16. Peterson GM, Nolan BW, Millingen KS. Survey of disability that is associated with Parkinson's disease. Med J Aust 1988;149:66,69-70.

17. Mutch WJ, Strudwick A, Roy SK, et al. Parkinson's disease: disability, review, and management. BMJ 1986;293:675-677.

18. Whetten-Goldstein K, Sloan F, Kulas E et al. The burden of Parkinson's disease on society, family, and the individual. JAGS 1977;45:844-849.

19. Carter JH, Stewart BJ, Archbold PG, et al. Living with a person who has Parkinson's disease: the spouse perspective by stage of disease. Mov Disord 1998;13:20-28.

20. King D, Playfer JR, Roberts NB. Concentrations of vitamins A, C, and E in elderly patients with Parkinson's disease. Postgrad med J 1992;68:634-637.

21. Carter JH, Nutt JG, Woodward WR. Amount and distribution of dietary protein affects clinical response to levadopa in Parkinson's disease. Neurology 1989;39:552-553.

REFERENCES

Chapter 1

1. Parkinson J. An essay on the shaking palsy. London; Sherwood, Neely & Jones 1817, 66.

2. Braak H, Ghebremedhin E, Rub U, et al. Stages in the development of Parkinson's disease-related pathology. Cell Tissue Res. 2004 Oct;318(1):121-34. Epub 2004 Aug 24.

3. Wendell CM, Hauser RA, Nagaria MH, Sanchez-Ramos J, Zesiewicz TA. Chief complaints of patients with Parkinson's disease. Neurology 1999;52(Suppl 2):A90.

4. Shulman LM, Taback RL, Rabinstein AA, Weiner WJ. Non-recognition of depression and other non-motor symptoms in Parkinson's disease.Parkinsonism Relat Disord. 2002 Jan;8(3):193-7.

5. Duvoisin RC. History of parkinsonism. Pharmacology and Therapeutics 1987;32:1-17.

6. Martilla RJ, Rinne UK. Epidemiological approaches to the etiology of Parkinson's disease. Acta Neurol Scand 1989;126:13-18.

7. Martilla RJ, Rinne UK. Epidemiology of Parkinson's disease in Finland. Acta Neurol Scand 1976; 53(2);81-102.

8. Lilienfeld DE, Chan E, Ehland J, Godbold J, Landrigan PH, Marsh G, Perl DP. Two decades of increasing mortality from Parkinson's disease among the US elderly. Arch Neurol 1990;47:731-734.

9. Tanner CM, Ben-Shlomo Y. Epidemiology of Parkinson's disease. Adv Neurol 1999;80:153-159.

10. Rajput AH, Offord K, Beard CM, Kurland LT. Epidemiology of Parkinsonism: incidence, classification, and mortality. Ann Neurol 1984;16:278-282.

11. Ben-Shlomo Y, Sieradzan K. Idiopathtic Parkinosn's disease: epidemiology, diagnosis, and management. Br. J Gen Pract 1995;45:261-268.

12. Bharucha NE, Bharucha EP, Bharucha AE, Bhise AV, Schoenberg BS. Prevalence of Parkinson's disease in the Parsi community of Bombay, India. Arch Neurol 1988;45:1321-1323.

13. Chan DK, Cordate D, Karr M, Ong B, Lei H, Liu J, Hung WT. Prevalence of Parkinson's disease in Sydney. Acta Neurol Scand 2005;111(1):7-11.

14. Melcon MO, Anderson DW, Vergara RH, Rocca WA. Prevalence of Parkinson's Disease in Junin, Buenos Aires Province, Argentina. Mov Disord 1997;12:197-205.

15. Morgante L, Rocca WA, DiRosa AE et al. Prevalence of Parkinson's disease and other types of parkinsonism: a door-to-door survey in three Sicilian municipalities. Neurology 1992;42:1901-1907.

16. Kessler II. Epidemiologic studies of Parkinson's disease. American J of Epi 1972;95:308-318.

17. Cosnett JE, Bill PL. Parkinson's disease in blacks. Observations on epidemiology in Natal. South African Medical Journal 1988;73:281-3.

18. Schoenberg BS, Anderson DW, Haerer AF. Prevalence of Parkinson's disease in the biracial population of Copiah County, Mississippi. Neurology 1985;35:841-845.

19. Mayeux R, Marder K, Cote L, Denaro J, Hemenegildo N, Mejia H, Tang MX, Lantigua R, Wilder D, Gurland B, Hauser A. The frequency of idiopathic Parkinson's disease by age, ethnic group, and sex in northern Manhattan, 1988-1993. Am J Epidemiol 1995;142:820-827.

20. Manyam BV. Paralysis agitans and levodopa in "Ayurveda": ancient Indian medical treatise. Movement Disorders 1990;5:47-8.

21. Ballard PA, Tetrud JW, Langston JW. Permanent human parkinsonism due to 1-methyl-4-phenyl-1,2,3,6-tetrahydropyridine (MPTP): seven cases. Neurology 1985;35:949-956.

22. Frigerio R, Elbaz A, Sanft KR, Peterson BJ, Bower JH, Ahlskog JE, Grossardt BR, de Andrade M, Maraganore DM, Rocca WA. Education and occupations preceding Parkinson disease: a population-based case-control study.Neurology. 2005 Nov 22;65(10):1575-83.

23. Hoehn MM. The natural history of Parkinson's disease in the pre-levodopa and post-levodopa eras. In: Cedarbaum JM, Gancher ST eds. Neurologic Clinics. Philadelphia PA: W.B. Saunders and Company 1992;331.

24. Tanner CM, Thelen JA, Offord KP, Rademacher D, Goetz CG, Kurland LT. Relationship of age at diagnosis to survival in Parkinson's disease (PD). Mov Disord 1992;7:104.

25. Diederich NJ, Moore CG, Leurgans SE, et al.Parkinson disease with old-age onset: a comparative study with subjects with middle-age onset. Arch Neurol. 2003 Apr;60(4):529-33.

26. Roos RA, Jongen JC, van der Velde EA.Clinical course of patients with idiopathic Parkinson's disease. Mov Disord. 1996 May;11(3):236-42.

27. Parashos SA, Maraganore DM, O'Brien PC, Rocca WA. Medical services utilization and prognosis in Parkinson disease: a population-based study. Mayo Clin Proc. 2002 Sep;77(9):918-25.

28. Wichman T, DeLong M. Pathophysiology of parkinsonian motor abnormalities. In: Narabayashi H, Nagatsu T, Yanagisawa N, Mizuno Y. Advances in Neurology New York: Raven Press 1993;53-60.

29. Gibb WRG. Neuropathology of movement disorders. J Neurol Neurosurg Psych 1989;55-67.

30. Hirsch E, Graybiel AM, Agid YA. Melanized dopaminergic neurons are differentially susceptible to degeneration in Parkinson's disease. Nature 1988;334:345-348.

31. Fearnley JM, Lees AJ. Ageing and Parkinson's disease: substantia nigra regional selectivity. Brain 1991;114:2283-2301.

32. Poewe WH, Wenning GK. The natural history of Parkinson's disease. Ann Neurol 1998; 44(Suppl 1):S1-S9.

33. Spillantini MG, Schmidt ML, Lee VM et al. Alpha-synuclein in Lewy bodies. Nature 1997; 388:839-840.

34. Richards M, Marder K, Cote L, Mayeux R. Reliability of symptom onset assessment in Parkinson's disease. Mov Disord 1994;9:340-342.

35. Aarsland D, Larsen JP, Lim NG, Janvin C, Karlsen D, Tandberg E, Cummings JL. Range of neuropsychiatric disturbances in patients with Parkinson's disease. J Neurol Neurosurg Psychiatry 1999;67:492-496.

36. Nagatsu T. Biochemical aspects of Parkinson's disease. In: Narabayashi H, Nagatsu T, Yanagisawa N, Mizuno Y. Advances in Neurology New York: Raven Press 1993;165-174.

37. Agid Y, Cervera P, Hirsch E, Javoy-Agid F, Lehericy S, Raisman R, Ruberg M. Biochemistry of Parkinson's disease 28 years later: a critical review. Movement Disorders 1989;4:S126-44.

38. Goldstein M, Lieberman A. The role of the regulatory enzymes of catecholamine synthesis in Parkinson's disease. Neurology 1992;42:8-12

39. Sibley DR, Monsma FJ Jr. Molecular biology of dopamine receptors. Trends Pharmacol Sci 1992;13:61-9.

40. Kebabian JW, Calne DB. Multiple receptors for dopamine. Nature 1979;277:93-96.

41. Calne DB. Treatment of Parkinson's disease. New Eng J Med 1993;3239:1021-1027.

42. Brooks DJ, Ibanez V, Sawle GV, et al. Differing patterns of striatal 18F-dopa uptake in Parkinson's disease, multiple system atrophy, and progressive supranuclear palsy.Ann Neurol 1990;28:547-55.

43. Brucke T, Kornhuber J, Angelberger P, Asenbaum S, Frassine H, Podreka I. SPECT imaging of dopamine and serotonin transporters with [123I] beta-CIT. Binding kinetics in the human brain. J Neurol Transm 1993;94:137-46.

Chapter 2

1. Marder K, Tang MX, Meijia H, et al. Risk of Parkinson's disease among first-degree relatives: a community-based study. Neurology 1996;47:155-160.

2. Lazzarini AM, Myers RH, Zimmerman TR Jr, et al. A clinical genetic study of Parkinson's disease: evidence for dominant transmission. Neurology 1994;44:499-506.

3. Ward CD, Duvoisin RC, Ince SE, et al. Parkinson's disease in 65 pairs of twins and in a set of quadruplets. Neurology 1983:33:815-824.

4. Tanner CM, Ottman R, Ellenberg JH et al. Parkinson's disease in twins: an etiologic study. JAMA 1999;281:341-346.

5. Piccini P, Burn DJ, Ceravolo R et al. The role of inheritance in sporadic Parkinson's disease: evidence from a longitudinal study of dopaminergic function in twins. Ann Neurol 1999;45:577-582.

6. Sveinbjornsdöttir S, Hicks AA, Jonsson T, et al. Familial aggregation of Parkinson's disease in Iceland. N Engl J Med. 2000;343:1765-1770.

7. Golbe LI, Di Iorio G, Sanges G et al. Clinical genetic analysis of Parkinson's disease in the Contursi kindred. Ann Neurol 1996;40:767-775.

8. Polymeropoulos MH, Higgins JJ, Golbe LI et al. Mapping of a gene for Parkinson's disease in the Contursi kindred. Science 1996;274:1265-1269.

9. Polymeropoulos MH, Lavedan C, Leroy E. Mutation in the a-synuclein gene identified in families with Parkinson's disease. Science 1997;276:2045-2047.

10. Markopoulou K, Wszolek ZK, Pfeiffer RF. A Greek-American kindred with autosomal dominant, levodopa-responsive parkinsonism and anticipation. Ann Neurol 1995;38:373-378.

11. Krüger R, Kuhn W, Muller T, et al. Ala30Pro mutation in the gene encoding alpha-synuclein in Parkinson's disease. Nat Genet 1998;18:106-108.

12. Zarranz JJ, Alegre J, Gomez-Esteban JC, et al. The new mutation, E46K, of alpha-synuclein causes Parkinson and Lewy body dementia. Ann Neurol 2004;55:164-173.

13. Singleton AB, Farrer M, Johnson J, et al. Alpha-Synuclein locus triplication causes Parkinson's disease. Science.2003;302:841.

14. Chartier-Harlin MC, Kachergus J, Roumier C, et al. Alpha-synuclein locus duplication as a cause of familial Parkinson's disease. Lancet 2004364:1167-1169.

15. Lee HJ, Patel S, Lee SJ. Intravesicular localization and exocytosis of alpha-synuclein and its aggregates. J Neurosci 2005;25:6016-6024.

16. Lashuel HA, Petre BM, Wall J, Simon M, Nowak RJ, Walz T, Lansbury PT Jr. Alpha-synuclein, especially the Parkinson's disease-associated mutants, forms pore-like annular and tubular protofibrils. J Mol Biol 2002;322:1089-1092.

17. Spillantini MG, Schmidt ML, Lee VM et al. Alpha-synuclein in Lewy bodies. Nature 1997;388:839-840.

18. Feany MB, Bender WW. A Drosophila model of Parkinson's disease. Nature 2000;404:394-398.

19. Lotharius J, Brundin P. Impaired dopamine storage resulting from alpha-synuclein mutations may contribute to the pathogenesis of Parkinson's disease. Hum Mol Genet 2002;11:2395-2407.

20. Conway KA, Rochet JC, Bieganski RM, Lansbury PT Jr. Kinetic stabilization of the alpha-synuclein protofibril by a dopamine-alpha-synuclein adduct. Science 2001;294:1346-1349.

21. Dauer W, Kholodilov N, Vila M, et al. Resistance of alpha -synuclein null mice to the parkinsonian neurotoxin MPTP. Proc Natl Acad Sci USA 2002;99:14524-14529.

22. Betarbet R, Sherer TB, MacKenzie G, Garcia-Osuna M, Panov AV, Greenamyre JT. Chronic systemic pesticide exposure reproduces features of Parkinson's disease. Nat Neurosci 2000;3:1301-1306.

23. Uversky VN, Li J, Bower K, Fink AL. Synergistic effects of pesticides and metals on the fibrillation of alpha-synuclein: implications for Parkinson's disease. Neurotoxicology 2002;23:527-536.

24. Auluck PK, Chan HY, Trojanowski JQ, Lee VM, Bonini NM. Chaperone suppression of alpha-synuclein toxicity in a Drosophila model for Parkinson's disease. Science 2002;295:865-868.

25. Auluck PK, Bonini NM. Pharmacological prevention of Parkinson disease in Drosophila. Nat Med 2002;8:1185-1186.

26. Arima K, Hirai S, Sunohara N, et al. Cellular co-localization of phosphorylated tau- and NACP/alpha-synuclein-epitopes in lewy bodies in sporadic Parkinson's disease and in dementia with Lewy bodies. Brain Res 1999;843:53-61.

27. Giasson BI, Forman MS, Higuchi M, et al. Initiation and synergistic fibrillization of tau and alpha-synuclein. Science 2003;300:636-640.

28. Ishikawa A, Tsuji S. Clinical analysis of 17 patients in 12 Japanese families with autosomal recessive type juvenile parkinsonism. Neurology 1996;47:160-166.

29. Kitada T, Asakawa H, Hattori N et al. Mutations in the parkin gene cause autosomal recessive juvenile parkinsonism. Nature 1998;392:605-608.

30. Lücking CB, Durr A, Bonifati V, et al. Association between early-onset Parkinson's disease and mutations in the parkin gene. French Parkinson's Disease Genetics Study Group. N Engl J Med. 2000;342:1560-1567.

31. West A, Periquet M, Lincoln S, et al. Complex relationship between Parkin mutations and Parkinson disease. Am J Med Genet 2002;114:584-591.

32. Oliveira SA, Scott WK, Martin ER, et al. Parkin mutations and susceptibility alleles in late-onset Parkinson's disease. Ann Neurol 2003;53:624-629.

33. Shimura H, Hattori N, Kubo S, et al. Familial Parkinson disease gene product, parkin, is a ubiquitin-protein ligase. Nat Genet 2000;25:302-305.

34. Tanaka K, Suzuki T, Chiba T, Shimura H, Hattori N, Mizuno Y. Parkin is linked to the ubiquitin pathway. J Mol Med 2001;79:482-494.

35. Bennett MC, Bishop JF, Leng, Chock PB, Chase TN, Mouradian MM. Degradation of alpha-synuclein by proteasome. J Biol Chem 1999;274:33855-33858.

36. Leroy E, Boyer R, Auburger G, et al. The ubiquitin pathway in Parkinson's disease. Nature 1998;395:451-452.

37. Maraganore DM, Lesnick TG, Elbaz A, et al. UCHL1 is a Parkinson's disease susceptibility gene. Ann Neurol 2004;55:512-521.

38. Valente EM, Abou-Sleiman PM, Caputo V, et al. Hereditary early-onset Parkinson's disease caused by mutations in PINK1. Science 2004;304:1158-1160.

39. Petit A, Kawarai T, Paitel E, et al. Wild-type PINK1 prevents basal and induced neuronal apoptosis, a protective effect abrogated by Parkinson disease-related mutations. J Biol Chem 2005;280:34025-34032.

40. Bonifati V, Rizzu P, van Baren MJ, et al. Mutations in the DJ-1 gene associated with autosomal recessive early-onset parkinsonism. Science 2003;299:256-259.

41. Junn E, Taniguchi H, Heong BS, Zhao X, Ichijo, Mouradian MM. Interaction of DJ-1 with Daxx inhibits apoptosis signal-regulating kinase 1 activity and cell death. Proc Natl Acad Sci USA 2005;102:9691-9696.

42. Paisan-Ruiz C, Jain S, Evans EW, et al. Cloning of the gene containing mutations that cause PARK8-linked Parkinson's disease. Neuron 2004;44:595-600.

43. Zimprich A, Biskup S, Leitner P, et al. Mutations in LRRK2 cause autosomal-dominant parkinsonism with pleomorphic pathology. Annn Neurol 2004;44:601-607.

44. Nichols WC, Pankratz N, Hernandez D, et al. Genetic screening for a single common LRRK2 mutation in familial Parkinson's disease. Lancet 2005;365:410-412.

45. Gasser T, Muller-Myhsok B, Wszolek ZK, et al. A susceptibility locus for Parkinson's disease maps to chromosome 2p13. Nature Genet 1998;18:262-265.

46. Karamohamed S, DeStefano AL, Wilk JB, et al. A haplotype at the PARK3 locus influences onset age for Parkinson's disease: the GenePD study. Neurology 2003;61:1557-1561.

47. Pankratz N, Uniacke SK, Halter CA, et al. Genes influencing Parkinson disease onset: replication of PARK3 and identification of novel loci. Neurology 2004;62:1616-1618.

48. DeStefano AL, Lew MF, Golbe LI, et al. PARK3 influences age at onset in Parkinson disease: a genome scan in the GenePD study. Am J Hum Genet 2002;70:1085-1089.

49. Hampshire D J, Roberts E, Crow Y, et al. Kufor-Rakeb syndrome, pallido-pyramidal degeneration with supranuclear upgaze paresis and dementia, maps to 1p36. J Med Genet 2001;38:680-682.

50. Hicks AA, Petursson H, Jonsson T, et al. A susceptibility gene for late-onset idiopathic Parkinson's disease. Ann Neurol 2002;52:549-555.

51. Pankratz N, Nichols WC, Uniacke SK, et al. Genome screen to identify susceptibility genes for Parkinson disease in a sample without parkin mutations. Am J Hum Genet 2002;71:124-135.

52. Pankratz N, Nichols WC, Uniacke SK, et al. Genome-wide linkage analysis and evidence of gene-by-gene interactions in a sample of 362 multiplex Parkinson disease families. Hum Molec Genet 2003;12: 2599-2608.

53. Farrer M, Maraganore DM, Lockhart P, et al. alpha-Synuclein gene haplotypes are associated with Parkinson's disease. Hum Mol Genet 2001;10:1847-1851.

54. Golbe LI, Lazzarini AM, Spychala JR, et al. The tau A0 allele in Parkinson's disease. Mov Disord 2001;16:442-447.

55. Menegon A, Board PG, Blackburn AC, Mellick GD, Le Couteur DG. Parkinson's disease, pesticides, and glutathione transferase polymorphisms. Lancet 1998;352:1344-1346.

56. Earle KM. Studies on Parkinson's disease including x-ray fluorescence spectroscopy of formalin-fixed brain tissue. J Neuropath Exp Neurol 1968;27:1-14.

57. Kim KS, Choi SY, Kwon HY, Won MH, Kang TC, Kang JH. Aggregation of alpha-synuclein induced by the Cu,Zn-superoxide dismutase and hydrogen peroxide system. Free Radic Biol Med 2002;32:544-550.

58. Hashimoto M, Hsu LJ, Xia Y, Takeda A, Sisk A, Sundsmo M, Masliah E. Oxidative stress induces amyloid-like aggregate formation of NACP/alpha-synuclein in vitro. Neuro Report 1999;10:717-721.

59. Sian J, Dexter DT, Lees AJ, et al. Alterations in glutathione levels in Parkinson's disease and other neurodegenerative disorders affecting basal ganglia. Ann Neurol 1994;36:348-355.

60. Gerlach M, Ben-Shachar D, Riederer P, Youdim MBH. Altered brain metabolism of iron as a cause of neurodegenerative diseases? J Neurochem 1994;63:793-807.

61. Youdim MB, Ben-Shachar D, Riederer P. The enigma of neuromelanin in Parkinson's disease substantia nigra. J Neurol Trans 1994;43:113-122.

62. Davis GC, Williams AC, Markey SP, Ebert MH, Caine ED, Reichert CM, Kopin IJ. Chronic parkinsonism secondary to intravenous injection of meperidine analogues. Psychiatry Research 1979;1:249-254.

63. Ballard PA, Tetrud JW, Langston JW. Permanent human parkinsonism due to 1-methyl-4-phenyl-1,2,3,6 tetrahydropyridine (MPTP): seven cases. Neurology 1985;35:949-956.

64. Semchuk KM, Love EJ, Lee RG. Parkinson's disease: a test of the multifactorial etiologic hypothesis. Neurology 1993;43:1173-1180.

65. Schapira AH, Mann VM, Cooper JM, et al. Anatomic and disease specificity of NADH CoQ1 reductase (complex 1) deficiency in Parkinson's disease. J Neurochem 1990;55:2142-2145.

66. Haas RH, Nsairian F, Nakano K, Ward D, Pay M, Hill R, Shults CW. Low platelet mitochondrial complex I and complex II/III activity in early untreated Parkinson's disease. Ann Neurol 1995;37:714-722.

67. Kessler II. Epidemiologic studies of Parkinson's disease. 3. A community-based survey. American Journal of Epidemiology 1972;96:242-254.

68. Hernan MA, Takkouche B, Caamano-Isorna F, Gestal-Otero JJ. A meta-analysis of coffee drinking, cigarette smoking, and the risk of Parkinson's disease. Ann Neurol 2002;52:276-284

69. Racette BA, Tabbal SD, Jennings D, Good L, Perlmutter JS, Evanoff B. Prevalence of parkinsonism and relationship to exposure in a large sample of Alabama welders. Neurology 2005;64:230-235.

70. Fearnley JM, Lees AJ. Aging and Parkinson's disease: substantia nigra regional selectivity. Brain 1991;114:2283-2301.

71. Neuman RP, LeWitt PA, Jaffe M, Calne DB, Larsen TA. Motor function in the normal aging population; treatment with levodopa. Neurology 1985;35:571-573.

72. Schwartz J, Elizan T. Search for viral particles and virus-specific products in idiopathic Parkinson's disease brain material. Ann Neurol 1979;6:261-263.

Chapter 3

1. Schou M, Baastrup PC, Grof P, Weis P, Angst J. Pharmacological and clinical problems of lithium prophylaxis. Br J Psych 1970;116:615-619.

2. Yamadori A, Albert M. Involuntary movement disorder caused by methyldopa. N Eng J Med 1972;286:610.

3. Rajput AH, Rozdilsky B, Hornykiewicz O et al. Reversible drug-induced parkinsonism. Arch Neurol 1982;39:644-646.

4. Logan WJ, Freeman JM. Pseudodegenerative disease due to diphenylhydantoin intoxication. Arch Neurol 1969;21:631-637.

5. Karas BJ, Wilder BJ, Hammond EJ et al. Treatment of valproate tremors. Neurology 1983;33:1380-1382.

6. Gibb WRG. Accuracy in the clinical diagnosis of parkinsonian syndromes. Postgraduate Med Jour 1988;64:345-351.

7. Ballard PA, Tetrud JW, Langston JW. Permanent human parkinsonism due to 1-methyl-4-phenyl-1,2,3,6-tetrahydropyridine (MPTP): seven cases. Neurology 1985;35:949-956.

8. Tolosa ES, Santamaria J. Parkinsonism and basal ganglia infarcts. Neurology 1984;34:1516-8.

9. Ferbert A, Gerwig M. Tremor due to stroke. Movement Disorders 1993;8:179-182.

10. Duvoisin RC, Yahr MD. Encephalitis and parkinsonism. Arch Neurol 1965;12:227-239.

11. Ziegler LH. Follow-up studies on persons who have had epidemic encephalitis. JAMA 1928;91:138-141.

12. Martland JS. Punch drunk. JAMA 1928;91:1103-7.

13. Corselis JAN, Bruton CJ, Freeman-Browne D. The aftermath of boxing. Psychol Med 1973;3:270-303.

14. Larsen TA, Calne DB. Essential tremor. Clin Neuropharmacol 1983;6:185-206.

15. Critchley M. Observations on essential (heredofamilial) tremor. Brain 1949;72:113-39.

16. Larson T, Sjogren T. Essential tremor. A clinical and genetic population study. Acta Psychiatr Neurol Scand 1960;36:1-176.

17. Koller WC, Busenbark K, Gray C, Hassanein RS, Dubinsky R. Classification of essential tremor. Clin Neurophar 1992;15:81-87.

18. Wilson SAK. Progressive lenticular degeneration: a familial nervous disease associated with cirrhosis of the liver. Brain 1912;34:295-507.

19. Levine IM, Estes JW, Looney JM. Hereditary neurological disease with acanthocytosis. A new syndrome. Arch Neurol 1968;19:403-409.

20. Aminoff MJ. Acanthocytosis and neurological disease. Brain 1972;95:749-760.

21. Sotaniemi KA. Chorea acanthocythosis-neurologic disease with acanthocytosis. Acta Neurol Scand 1983;68:53-56.

22. Huntington G. On Chorea. Lea and Blanchard, Philadelphia, Medical and Surgical Reporter 1872;26:317.

23. Hayden MR. Huntington's chorea. New York, Springer-Verlag, 1981.

24. Huntington's Disease Collaborative Research Group. A novel gene containing a trinucleotide repeat that is expanded and unstable on Huntington's disease chromosomes. Cell 1993;72:971-983.

25. Klawans HL, Weiner WJ. The pharmacology of choreatic movement disorder. Prog Neurobiol 1976;6:49-80.

26. Steele JC, Richardson JC, Olszewski J. Progressive supranuclear palsy. Arch Neurol 1964;10:333-359.

27. Golbe LI, Davis PH, Schoenberg BS, Duvoisin RC. Prevalence and natural history of progressive supranuclear palsy. Neurology 1988;38:1031-1034.

28. Jankovic J, Friedman DI, Pirozzolo FJ, McCrary JA. Progressive supranuclear palsy: motor, neurobehavioral, and neuro-ophthalmic findings.In: Streifler MB, Korczyn AD, Melamed E, Youdim MBH, Advances in Neurology; Raven Press, New York, 1990.

29. Fukushima- Kudo J, Fukushima K, Tashiro K. Rigidity and dorsiflexion of the neck inprogressive supranuclear palsy and the interstitial nucleus of Cajal. J Neurol Neurosurg Psychiatry 1987;50:1197-1203.

30. Pillon B, Dubois B, Lhermitte F, Agid Y. Heterogeneity of cognitive impairment in progressive supranuclear palsy, Parkinson's disease, and Alzheimer's disease. Neurology 1986;36:1179-1185.

31a. Oppenheimer DR. Diseases of the basal ganglia, cerebellum and motorneurons. In Blackwood W, Corsellis JAN Eds: Greenfield's Neuropathology. London, Edward Arnold 1976:608-651.

31b. Quinn N. Multiple system atrophy-the nature of the beast. J Neurol Neurosurg Psychiatry 1989;52:78-79.

32. Colosimo C, Riple D, Wenning GK. Management of multiple system atrophy: state of the art. J Neural Transm 2005;112:1695-1704.

33. Shy GM, Drager GA. A neurological syndrome associated with orthostatic hypotension: a clinical-pathological study. Arch Neurol 1960;2:511-527.

34. Rajput AH, Rozdilsky B. Dysautonomia in parkinsonism: a clinicopathological study. J Neurol Neurosurg Psychiatry 1976;39:1092-1100.

35. Lees AJ, Bannister R. The use of lisuride in the treatment of multiple system atrophy with autonomic failure (Shy-Drager syndrome). J Neurol Neurosurg Psychiatry 1981;44:347-351.

36. Dejerine J, Thomas A. L'atrophie olivo-ponto-cerebelleuses. Nouv Iconogr Salpet 1900; 13:330-370.

37. Berciano J. Olivopontocerebellar atrophy. J Neurol Sci 1982;53:253-272.

38. Koeppen AH, Barron KD. The neuropathology of olivopontocerebellar atrophy. In: Duvoisin RC, Plaitakis A Eds: The Olivopontocerebellar Atrophies. New York, Raven Press 1984:13-38.

39. Huang YP, Plaitakis A. Morphological changes of olivoponto cerebellar atrophy in computed tomography and comments on its pathogenesis. In Duvoisin RC, Plaitakis A Eds: The Olivopontocerebellar Atrophies. New York, Raven Press 1984:39-85.

40. Adams RD, Van Bogaert L, Van Der Eecken H. Striatonigral degeneration. J Neuropath Exp Neurol 1964;23:584-608.

41. Takei Y, Samuels NS. Striatonigral degeneration: a form of multiple system atrophy with clinical parkinsonism. In: Zimmerman HM Ed: Progress in Neuropathology Vol 2 New York, Grune and Stratton 1973, 217-251.

42. Reibeiz JJ, Kolodny EH, Richardson E. Corticodentatonigral degeneration with neuronal achromasia. Arch Neurol 1968;18:20-33.

43. Riley DE, Lang AE, Lewis A, et al. Cortical-basal ganglionic degeneration. Neurology 1990;40:1203-1212.

44. Case records of the Massachusetts General Hospital. N Engl J Med 1985;313:739-748.

45. Louis ED, Goldman JE, Powers JM, Fahn S. Parkinsonian features of eight pathologically diagnosed cases of diffuse Lewy body disease. Movement Disorders 1994;10:188-94.

46. Hansen LA, Galasko D. Lewy body disease. Current Opinion in Neurology & Neurosurgery. 1992;5:889-94.

Chapter 4

1. Calne DB, Stoessl AJ. Early parkinsonism. Clinical Neuropharmacology 1986;9:S3-8.

2. Calne DB, Snow BJ, Lee C. Criteria for diagnosing Parkinson's disease. Ann Neurol 1992;32:S125-127.

3. Martilla RJ, Rinne UK. Epidemiology of Parkinson's disease in Finland. Acta Neurol Scand 1976;53:81-102.

4. Gudmundsson KRA. A clinical survey of parkinsonism in Iceland. Acta Neurol Scand 1967;43(suppl):9-61.

5. Nobrega FT, Glattre E, Kurland LT, Okazaki H. Comments on the epidemiolgy of parkinsonism including prevalence and incidence statistics for Rochester, Minnesota, 1935-1966. In: Barbeau A, Brunette JR, eds. Progress in Neurogenetics. Proceedings of the Second International Congress of Neurogenetics and Neuro-Ophthalmology. Amsterdam: Excerpta Medica, 1969.

6. Litvan I, Bhatia KP, Burn DJ, Goetz CG, Lang AE, McKeith I, Quinn N, Sethi KD, Shults C, Wenning GK; Movement Disorders Society Scientific Issues Committee. Movement Disorders Society Scientific Issues Committee report: SIC Task Force appraisal of clinical diagnostic criteria for Parkinsonian disorders. Mov Disord. 2003 May;18(5):467-86.

7. Daniel SE, Lees AJ. Parkinson's Disease Society Brain Bank, London: overview and research. J Neural Transm Suppl. 1993;39:165-72.

8. Gibb WRG, Lees AJ. The clinical phenomenon of akathisia. J Neur Neurosurg Psych 1986;49:861-866.

9. Hoehn MM, Yahr MD. Parkinsonism: onset, progression and mortality. Neurology 1967;17: 427-442.

10. Mutch WJ, Dingwall-Fordyce I, Downie AW, Paterson JG, Roy SK. Parkinson's disease in a Scottish city. Br Med J 1986;292:534-536.

11. Schrag A, Ben-Shlono Y, Brown R, Marsden CD, Quinn N. Young-onset Parkinson's disease revisited - clinical features, natural history, and mortality. Mov Disord 1998;13:885-894.

12. Rosati G, Granieri E, Pinna L, et al. The risk of Parkinson's disease in Mediterranean people. Neurology 1980;30:250-255.

13. Harada H, Nishikawa S, Takahaski K. Epidemiology of Parkinson's disease in a Japanese city. Arch Neurol 1983;40:151-154.

14. Gibb WRG, Lees AJ. A comparison of clinical and pathological features of young-and old-onset Parkinson's disease. Neurology 1988;38:1402-1406.

15. Aarsland D, Larsen JP, Lim NG, et al. Range of neuropsychiatric disturbnaces in patients with Parkinson's disease. J Neurol Neurosurg Psychiatry 1999;67:492-496.

16. Juncos JL. Management of psychotic aspects of Parkinson's disease. J Clin Psychiatry 1999;60 (suppl 8): 42-53.

17. Cummings JL. Behavioral complications of drug treatment of Parkinson's disease. J Am Geriatr Soc 1991;39:708-716.

18. Factor SA, Molho ES, Podskalny GD, et al. Parkinson's disease: drug-induced psychiatric states. Adv Neurol 1995;65:115-138.

19. Hoehn M. Commentary: Parkinsonism: onset, progression, and mortality. Neurology 1998;50(8):38.

20. Poewe WH, Wenning GK. The natural history of Parkinson's disease. Ann Neurol 1998;44 (Suppl 1):S1-S9.

21. Goetz CG, Movement Disorder Society Task Force report on the Hoehn and Yahr staging scale: status and recommendations. Mov Disord 2004;19:1020-1028.

22. Fahn S, Elton RL, Members of the UPDRS Development Committee. Unified Parkinson's disease rating scale. In: Fahn S, Marsden CD, Calne DB, Goldstein M, Eds. Recent developments in Parkinson's disease. Vol 2. Florham Park, NJ: Macmillan Health Care Information 1987, 153-164.

23. Movement Disorder Society Task Force on Rating Scales for Parkinson's Disease. The Unified Parkinson's Disease Rating Scale (UPDRS): Status and Recommendations. Mov Disord 2003;18: 738-750.

24. Schwab RS, England AC Jr. Projection techniques for evaluating surgery in Parkinson's Disease. pp 152-157 (Table 1, page 153). IN: Third Symposium on Parkinson's Disease, Royal College of Surgeons in Edinburgh, May 20-22, 1968. E&S Livingstone Ltd. 1969.

Chapter 5

1.   Fahn S. "On-off" phenomenon with levodopa therapy in parkinsonism. Clinical and pharmacologic correlates and the effect of intramuscular pyridoxine. Neurology 1974;24:431-441.

2.   Marsden CD, Parkes JD. "On-off" effects in patients with Parkinson's disease on chronic levodopa therapy. Lancet 1976;1:292-296.

3.   Sage JI, Mark M. The rationale for continuous dopaminergic stimulation in patients with Parkinson's disease (review). Neurology 1992;42:S23-8

4.   Chase TN, Mouradian MM, Engber TM. Motor response complications and the function of striatal efferent systems. Neurology 1993;43:S23-27.

5.   Muenter MD, Sharpless NS, Tyce GM, Darly FL. Patterns of dystonia ("I-D-I" and "D-I-D in response to L-dopa therapy for Parkinson's disease. Mayo Clin. Proc 1977;52:163-174.

6.   Mones RJ, Elizan TS, Siegel GJ. Analysis of L-dopa induced dyskinesias in 51 patients with parkinsonism. J Neurol Neurosurg Psychiatry 1971;34:668-73.

7.   McHale DM, Sage JI, Sonsalla PK, Vitagliano D. Complex dystonia of Parkinson's disease: clinical features and relation to plasma levodopa profile. Clinical Neuropharmacology 1990;13:164-170.

8.   Poewe WH, Lees AJ, Stern GM. Low-dose L-dopa therapy in Parkinson's disease; a six-year follow up. Neurology 1986;36:1528-1530.

9.   Hauser RA, Zesiewicz TA, Factor SA, Guttman M, Weiner W. Clinical trials of add-on medications in Parkinson's disease: efficacy versus usefulness. Parkinsonism Rel Disord 1997;3:1-6.

10.   Jenner P, Al-Barghouthy G, Smith L, et al. Initiation of entacapone with I-dopa further improves antiparkinsonian activity and avoids dyskinesia in the MPTP primate model of Parkinson's disease. Neurology 2002;58 (suppl 3):A374-A375.

11.   Pearce RK, Banerji T, Jenner P, Marsden CD. De novo administration of ropinirole and bromocriptine induces less dyskinesia than levodopa in MPTP-treated marmosets. Mov Disord 1998;13:234-241.

12.   Rascol O, Brooks DJ, Korczyn AD, et al. A five-year study of the incidence of dyskinesia in patients with early Parkinson's disease who were treated with ropinirole or levodopa. N Engl J Med 2000;342:1484-1491.

13.   Parkinson Study Group. Pramipexole versus levodopa as initial treatment for Parkinson's disease: a randomized controlled trial. JAMA 2000;284:1931-1938.

14.   Giladi N, McMahon D, Przedborski S, Flaster E, Guillory S, Kostic V, Fahn S. Motor blocks in Parkinson's disease. Neurology 1992;42:333-339.

15.   Witjas T, Kaphan E, Azulay JP, et al. Nonmotor fluctuations in Parkinson's disease: frequent and disabling. Neurology 2002;59:408-413.

16.   Stacy M, Bowron A, Guttman M, et al. Identification of motor and non-motor wearing-off in Parkinson's disease: Comparison of a patient questionnaire versus a clinician assessment. Mov Disord 2005;20:726-733.

Chapter 6

1.   Cotzias GC, Van Woert MH, Shiffer LM. Aromatic amino acids and modification of parkinsonism. N Engl J Med 1967;276:347-379.

2.   Carlsson A. The occurrence, distribution, and physiological role of catecholamines in the nervous system. Pharmacol Rev 1959;11:490-493.

3. Ehringer, H, Hornykiewicz O. Vertelung von noradrenalin and dopamin (3-hydroxytyramin) im gehirn des menschen und ihr verhalten bei erkrankum gen des extrapyramidalen systems. Klin Wschr 1960;38:1236-1239.

4. Cotzias GC, Papavasilou PS, Gellene R. Experimental treatment of parkinsonism with L-dopa. Neurology 1968;18:276-7.

5. Bartholini GJ, Pletscher A. Effects of various decarboxylase inhibitors on the cerebral metabolism of dihydroxyphenylalanine. J Pharamacol 1969;21:323-324.

6. Kurlan R, Rothfield AB, Woodward WR, Nutt JG, Miller C, Lichter D, and Shoulson I. Erratic gastric empyting of levodopa may cause "random" fluctuations of parkinsonian mobility. Neurology 1988;48:419-421.

7. Leon AS, Spiegel HE. The effect of antacid administration on the absorption and metabolism of levodopa. J Clinical Pharmacol 1972;12:263-267.

8. Nutt JG, Fellman JH. Pharmacokinetics of levodopa. Clin Neuropharm 1984;7:35-49.

9. Physicians Desk Reference 57th ed. Thompson PDR: Montvale, New Jersey, 2003.

10. Pahwa R, Lyons K, Marjama J, et al. Clinical experience with generic carbidopa/levodopa (G-L) in patients with Parkinson's disease. Neurology 1994;44(suppl 2):A244.

11. Pahwa R, Marjama J, McGuire D, et al. Pharmacokinetic comparison of Sinemet and Atamet (generic carbidopa/levodopa) a single dose study. Mov Disord 1996;11:427-430.

12. Pittner H, Stormann H, Enzenhofer R. Pharmacodynamic actions of midodrine, a new a-adrenergic stimulating agent, and its main metabolite, ST 1059. Arzneim Forsch 1976;26:2145-2154.

13. Goetz CG, Tanner CM, Klawans HL et al. Parkinson's disease and motor fluctuations: long-acting carbidopa/levodopa (CR4-Sinemet). Neurology 1987;37:875-878.

14. Yeh KC, August TF, Bush DF et al. Pharmacokinetics and bioavailability of Sinemet CR:a summary of human studies. Neurology 1989;39:S25-32.

15. Hutton JT, Morris JL. Long-acting carbidopa-levodopa in the management of moderate and advanced Parkinson's disease. Neurology 1992;42:51-56.

16. Rodnitzky R. The use of Sinemet CR in the management of mild to moderate Parkinson's disease. Neurology 1992;42 (suppl 1):44-50.

17. Brooks DJ, Agid Y, Eggert K, et al. Treatment of end-of-dose wearing-off in parkinson's disease: stalevo (levodopa/carbidopa/entacapone) and levodopa/DDCI given in combination with Comtess/Comtan (entacapone) provide equivalent improvements in symptom control superior to that of traditional levodopa/DDCI treatment. Eur Neurol. 2005;53(4):197-202.Epub 2005 Jun 20.

18. Myllylä V, Kaakkola S, Miettinen T, et al. New triple combination of levodopa/carbidopa/entacapone is a preferred treatment in patients with Parkinson's disease. Neurology 2003;60 (Suppl 1):A289.

19. Hauser RA. Levodopa/carbidopa/entacapone triple combination (Stalevo). Neurology 2004;62 (Suppl1):S64-71.

20. Block G, Liss C, Reines S, Irr J, Nibbelink D, The CR First Study Group. Comparison of immediate-release and controlled release carbidopa/levodopa in Parkinson's disease. A multi-center five-year study. Eur Neurol 1997;37:23-27.

21. Jenner P, Al-Barghouthy G, Smith L, et al. Initiation of entacapone with l-dopa further improves antiparkinsonian activity and avoids dyskinesia in the MPTP primate model of Parkinson's disease. Neurology 2002;58 (suppl 3):A374-A375.

22. Lees AJ. Madopar HBS (hydrodynamically balanced system) in the treatment of Parkinson's disease. In: Korczyn AD, Melamed E, Youdim MBH eds. Advances in Neurology New York: Raven Press, 1990:475-82.

23. Axelrod J, Senoh S, Witkop B. O-methylation of catecholamines in vivo. J Biol Chem 1958;233:697-701.

24. Guldberg HC, Marsden CA. Catechol-O-methyl transferase: pharmacological aspects and physiological role. Pharmacol Rev 1975;27:135-206.

25. Nissenen E, Tuominen R, Perhoniemi V, Kaakkola S. Catechol-O-methyltransferase activity in human and rat small intestine. Life Sci 1988;42:2609-2614.

26. Kastner A, Anglade P, Bounaix C, Damier P, Javoy-Agid F et al. Immunohistochemical study of catechol-O-methyltransferase in the human mesostriatal system. Neuroscience 1994;62:449-457.

27. Reeches A, Meilke LR, Fahn S. 3-O-methyldopa inhibits rotations induced by levodopa in rats after unilateral destruction of the nigrostriatal pathway. Neurology 1982;32:887-888.

28. Nutt JG, Woodward WR, Gancher ST, Merrick D. 3-O-methyldopa and the response to levodopa in Parkinson's disease. Ann Neurol 1987;21:584-588.

29. Kaakkola S, Wurtman RJ. Effects of catechol-O-methyltransferase inhibitors and L-3,4-dihydroxyphenylalanine with or without carbidopa on extracellular dopamine in rat striatum. J Neurochem 1993;60:137-144.

30. Kaakkola S, Teravainen H, Ahtila S, Rita H, Gordin A. Effect of entacapone, a COMT inhibitor, on clinical disability and levodopa metabolism in parkinsonism patients. Neurology 1994;44:77-80.

31. Keranen T, Gordin A, Harjola VP, Karlsson M, Lorpela K. The effect of catechol-O-methyl transferase inhibition by entacapone on the pharmacokinetics and metabolism of levodopa in healthy volunteers. Clin Neuropharm 1993;16:145-156.

32. Rinne UK, Gordin A, Teravainen H. COMT inhibition with entacapone in the treatment of Parkinson's diseases. Ann Neurol 1999;80:491-494.

33. Parkinson Study Group. Entacapone improves motor fluctuation in levodopa-treated Parkinson's disease patients. Ann Neurol 1997;42:747-755.

34. Rinne UK, Larsen JP, Siden A, Worm-Petersen J. Entacapone enhances the response to levodopa in parkinsonian patiens with motor fluctuations. Nomecomt Study Group. Neurology 1998;51:1309-1314.

35. Larsen JP and the NOMESAFE study group. Poster, ICPDMD, 2001.

36. Poewe WH, Deuschl G, Gordin A, et al. Efficacy and safety of entacapone in Parkinson's disease patients with suboptimal levodopa response: a six-month randomized placebo-controlled double-blind study in Germany and Austria (Celomen study). Acta Neurol Scand. 2002 Apr;105(4):245-55.

37. Onofrj M, Thomas A, Vingerhoets F, et al. Combining entacapone with levodopa/DDCI improves clinical status and quality of life in Parkinson's Disease (PD) patients experiencing wearing-off, regardless of the dosing frequency: results of a large multicentre open-label study. J Neural Transm 2004;111(8):1053-1063.

38. Stocchi F, Barbato L, Nordera G, et al. Entacapone improves the pharmacokinetic and therapeutic response of controlled release levodopa/carbidopa in Parkinson's patients. J Neural Transm. 2004 Feb;111(2):173-80

39. Olanow CW, Kieburtz K, Stern M, et al. Double-blind, placebo-controlled study of entacapone in levodopa-treated patients with stable Parkinson disease. Arch Neurol. 2004 Oct;61(10):1563-8.

40. Olanow CW, Stocchi F. COMT inhibitors in Parkinson's disease: can they prevent and/or reverse levodopa-induced motor complications? Neurology. 2004 Jan 13;62(1 Suppl 1):S72-81.

41. Smith LA, Jackson MJ, Al-Barghouthy G, Rose S, Kuoppamaki M, Olanow W, Jenner P. Multiple small doses of levodopa plus entacapone produce continuous dopaminergic stimulation and reduce dyskinesia induction in MPTP-treated drug-naive primates. Mov Disord. 2005 Mar;20(3):306-14.

42. Kaakkola S, Wurtman RJ. Effects of catechol-O-methyltransferase inhibitors and L-3, 4-dihydroxyphenylalanine with or without carbidopa on extracellular dopamine in rat striatum. J Neurochem 1993;60:137-144.

43. Dingemanse J, Jorga K, Zurcher G, Schmitt M, Sedek G et al. Pharmokinetic-pharmacodynamic interaction between the COMT inhibitor tolcapone and single-dose levodopa. Br J Clin Pharmacol 1995;40:253-262.

44. Waters CH, Kurth M, Bailey P, et al. Tolcapone in stable Parkinson's disease: efficacy and safety of long-term treatment. The Tolcapone Stable Study Group. Neurology 1997;49:665-671.

45. Rajput AH, Martin W, Saint-Hilaire MH, Dorflinger E, Pedder S. Tolcapone improves motor function in parkinsonian patients with the "wearing-off" phenomenon: a double-blind, placebo-controlled, multi-center trial. Neurology 1997;49:1066-1071.

46. Adler CH, Singer C, O'Brien C et al for the Tolcapone Study Group. Randomized, placebo-controlled study of tolcapone in patients with fluctuating Parkinson's disease treated with levodopa/carbidopa. Arch Neurol 1998;55:1089-1095.

47. Assal F, Spahr L, Hadengue A et al. Tolcapone and fulminant hepatitis. Lancet 1998;352:958.

48. Jenner P. The rationale for the use of dopamine agonists in Parkinson's disease. Neurology 1995;45:S6-12.

49. Montastruc, JL, Rascol O, Senard JM. Current status of dopamine agonists in Parkinson's disease management. Drugs 1993;46:384-393.

50. Langtry J, Clissold SP. Pergolide: a review of its pharmacological properties and therapeutic potential in Parkinson's disease. Drugs 1990;39:491-506.

51. Pritchett AM, Morrison JF, Edwards WD, Schaff HV, Connolly HM, Espinoza RE. Valvular heart disease in patients taking pergolide. Mayo Clinic Proc 2002;77:1280-1286.

52. Olanow CW, Fahn S, Muenter M. A multi-center double-blind placebo-controlled trial of pergolide as an adjunct to Sinemet in Parkinson's disease. Movement Disorders 1994;9:40-47.

53. Oertel WH, Wolters E, Sampaio C, et al. Pergolide versus levodopa monotherapy in early Parkinson's disease patients: The PELMOPET study Mov Disord. 2005 Oct 6.

54. Waller EA, Kaplan J, Heckman MG. Related Articles, Links Valvular heart disease in patients taking pergolide. Mayo Clin Proc. 2005 Aug;80 (8):1016-20.

55. Baseman DG, O'Suilleabhain PE, Reimold SC, et al. Pergolide use in Parkinson disease is associated with cardiac valve regurgitation. Neurology. 2004 Jul 27;63(2):301-4.

56. Horowski R, Jahnichen S, Pertz HH. Fibrotic valvular heart disease is not related to chemical class but to biological function: 5-HT2B receptor activation plays crucial role. Mov Disord. 2004 Dec;19(12):1523-4.

57. Comella CL, Morrissey M, Janko K. Nocturnal activity with nighttime pergolide in Parkinson disease: a controlled study using actigraphy. Neurology. 2005 Apr 26;64 (8):1450-1.

58. Brefel C, Thalamus C, Rayet S, et al. Effect of food on the pharmacokinetics of ropinirole in parkinsonian patients. Br J Clin Pharmacol 1998:45:412-415.

59. Kreider M, Knox S, Gardiner D, Wheadon D. A multi-center double-blind study of ropinirole as an adjunct to L-dopa in Parkinson's disease. Neurology 1996;46 (Suppl):A475.

60. Wheadon DE, Wilson-Lynch K, Gardiner D, Kreider MS. Ropinirole, a non-ergoline D2 agonist, is effective in early parkinsonian patients not treated with L-dopa. Movement Disorders 1996;11(Suppl 1):162.

61. Rascol O on behalf of the Study Group. A double-blind L-dopa controlled study of ropinirole in de novo patients with Parkinson's disease. Mov Disord 1996;11 (Suppl 1):139.

62. Rascol O, Brooks DJ, Korczyn AD, et al. A five-year study of the incidence of dyskinesia in patients with early Parkinson's disease who were treated with ropinirole or levodopa. N Engl J Med 2000;342:1484-1491.

63. Whone AL, Remy P, Davis MR, et al. The REAL-PET study: slower progression in early Parkinson's disease treated with ropinirole compared with l-dopa. Neurology 2002;58 (suppl 3):A82-A83.

64. Ling ZD, Robie HC, Tong CW, Carvey PM. Both the antioxidant and D3 agonist actions of pramipexole mediate its neuroprotective actions in mesencephalic cultures. J Pharmacol Exp Ther 1999;289:202-210.

65. Shannon KM, Bennett JP Jr, Friedman JH. Efficacy of pramipexole, a novel dopamine agonist, as monotherapy in mild to moderate Parkinson's disease. The Pramipexole Study Group. Neurology 1997;49:724-728.

66. Lieberman A, Ranhosky A, Korts D. Clinical evaluation of pramipexole in advanced Parkinson's disease: results of a double-blind, placebo-controlled, parallel-group study. Neurology 1997;49:162-168.

67. Weiner WJ, Factor SA, Jankovic J, et al. The long-term safety and efficacy of pramipexole in advanced Parkinson's disease. Parkinsonism Rel Disord 2001;7:115-120.

68. Parkinson Study Group. Pramipexole versus levodopa as initial treatment for Parkinson's disease: a randomized controlled trial. JAMA 2000;284:1931-1938.

69. Parkinson Study Group. Dopamine transporter brain imaging to assess the effects of pramipexole versus levodopa on Parkinson's disease progression. JAMA 2002;287: 1653-1661.

70. Pontiroli AE. Inhibition of basal and metoclopramide-induced prolactin release by cabergoline, an extremely long-acting dopaminergic drug. J Clin Endocrinol Metab 1987;65:1057-1059.

71. Ferrari C, Barbieri C, Caldara R, et al. Long-lasting prolactin lowering effect of cabergoline, a new dopamine agonist, in hyperprolactinemic patients. J Clin Endocrinol Met 1986;63:941-945.

72. Ahlskog JE, Muenter MD, Maraganore DM, Matsumoto JY, Lieberman A. Fluctuating Parkinson's disease:treatment with long-acting dopamine agonist cabergoline. Arch Neurol 1994;51: 1236-1241.

73. Hutton JT, Morris JL, Brewer MA. Controlled study of the antiparkinsonian activity and tolerability of cabergoline. Neurology 1993;43:613-616.

74. Bracco F, Battaglia A, Chouza C, et al. The long-acting dopamine receptor agonist cabergoline in early Parkinson's disease: final results of a 5-year, double-blind, levodopa-controlled study. CNS Drugs. 2004;18(11):733-46.

75. Townsend M, MacIver DH. Constrictive pericarditis and pleuropulmonary fibrosis secondary to cabergoline treatment for Parkinson's disease. Heart. 2004 Aug;90(8):e47.

76. Dhawan V, Medcalf P, Stegie F, et al. Retrospective evaluation of cardio-pulmonary fibrotic side effects in symptomatic patients from a group of 234 Parkinson's disease patients treated with cabergoline. J Neural Transm. 2005 May;112(5):661-8. Epub 2005 Mar 23.

77. Tyne HL, Parsons J, Sinnott A, et al. A 10 year retrospective audit of long-term apomorphine use in Parkinson's disease. J Neurol. 2004 Nov;251(11):1370-4.

78. Schwab RS, Amador LV, Lettvin JY. Apomorphine in Parkinson's disease. Trans Am Neurol Assoc. 1951;56:251-3.

79. Dewey Jr RB. 10 questions about using apomorphine for Parkinson disease. Neurologist. 2005 May;11(3):190-2.

80. Barker R, Duncan J, Lees AJ. Subcutaneous apomorphine as a diagnostic test for dopaminergic responsiveness in parkinsonian syndromes. Lancet 1989;1:675.

81. Dewey RB Jr, Hutton JT, LeWitt PA, et al. A randomized, double-blind, placebo-controlled trial of subcutaneously injected apomorphine for parkinsonian off-state events. Arch Neurol. 2001 Sep;58(9):1385-92.

82. Gopinathan G, Teravainen H, Dambrosia JM. Lisuride in parkinsonism. Neurology 1981;31:371-376.

83. Obeso JA, Luquin MR, Martinez J. Intravenous lisuride corrects oscillations of motor performance in Parkinson's disease. Ann Neurol 1986;19:31-35.

84. Obeso JA, Luquin MR, Vaamonde J, et al. Subcutaneous administration of lisuride in the treatment of complex motor fluctuations in Parkinson's disease. J Neurol Trans 1988;27:S17-25.

85. Montastruc JL, Rascol O, Senard JM, Rascol A. A randomised controlled study comparing bromocriptine to which levodopa was later added, with levodopa alone in previously untreated patients with Parkinson's disease: a five year follow up. Jour Neurol Neurosurg Psych 1994;57:1034-1038.

86. Hely MA, Morris JGL, Reid WGJ, O'Sullivan DJ, Williamson PM. The Sydney Multicentre Study of Parkinson's Disease: a randomized, prospective five year study comparing low-dose bromocriptine with low dose levodopa-carbidopa. Jour Neurol Neurosurg Psych 1994;57: 903-910.

87. Rinne UK. Early dopamine agonist therapy in Parkinson's disease. Movement Disorders 1989;4:S86-94.

88. Frucht S, Rogers JD, Greene PE, et al. Falling asleep at the wheel: motor vehicle mishaps in persons taking pramipexole and ropinirole. Neurology 1999;52:1908-1910.

89. Hobson DE, Lang AE, Martin WR, Razmy A, Rivest J, Fleming J. Excessive daytime sleepiness and sudden onset sleep in Parkinson's disease; a survey by the Canadian Movement Disorders Group. JAMA 2002;287:455-463.

90. Ondo WG, Dat Wong K, Kahn H, Atassi F, Kwak C, Jankovic J. Daytime sleepiness and other sleep disorders in Parkinson's disease. Neurology 2001;57:1392-1396.

91. Driver-Dunckley E, Samanta J, Stacy M. Pathological gambling associated with dopamine agonist therapy in Parkinson's disease. Neurology. 2003 Aug 12;61(3):422-3.

92. Dodd ML, Klos KJ, Bower JH, Geda YE, Josephs KA, Ahlskog JE. Pathological gambling caused by drugs used to treat Parkinson disease. Arch Neurol. 2005 Sep;62(9):1377-81

93. Klos KJ, Bower JH, Josephs KA, Matsumoto JY, Ahlskog JE. Pathological hypersexuality predominantly linked to adjuvant dopamine agonist therapy in Parkinson's disease and multiple system atrophy. Parkinsonism Relat Disord. 2005 Sep;11(6):381-6

94. Nirenberg MJ, Waters C. Related Articles, Links Compulsive eating and weight gain related to dopamine agonist use. Mov Disord. 2005 Oct 31; [Epub ahead of print]

95. Laine K, Anttila M, Heinonen E, et al. Lack of adverse interactions between concomitantly administered selegiline and citalopram. Clinical Neuropharmacology 1997;20:419-433.

96. Golbe LI. long-term efficacy and safety of deprenyl in advanced Parkinson's disease. Neurology 1989;39:1109-1111.

97. Birkmayer W, Riederer P, Youdim MBH et al. The potentiation of the anti-akinetic effect after L-dopa treatment by an inhibitor of MAO-B, Deprenil. J Neural Transm 1975;36:303-326.

98. Bodner RA, Lynch T, Lewis L, Kahn D. Serotonin syndrome. Neurology 1995;45:219-23.

99. Waters, C. Fluoxetine and selegiline-lack of significant interaction. Canadian Journal of Neurological Sciences 1994;21:259-261.

100. Parkinson Study Group. Effects of tocopherol and deprenyl on the progression of disability in early Parkinson's disease. N Engl J Med 1993;328:176-183.

101. Heikila RE, Manzino L, Cabbat FS, et al. Protection against the dopaminergic neurotoxicity of 1-methyl-4-phenyl-1,2,5,6-tetrahydropyridine by monoamine oxidase inhibitors. Nature 1984;311:467-469.

102. Parkinson Study Group. Effects of tocopherol and deprenyl on the progression of disability in early Parkinson's disease. N Engl J Med 1993;328:176-183.

103. Waters CH, Sethi KD, Hauser RA, et al. Zydis selegiline reduces off time in Parkinson's disease patients with motor fluctuations: a 3-month, randomized, placebo-controlled study. Mov Disord. 2004 Apr;19(4):426-32.

104. Finberg JP, Tenne M, Youdim MB. Tyramine antagonists properties of AGN 1130: an irreversible inhibitor of monoamine oxidase type B. Br J Pharamcol 1981;73:65-74.

105. Rascol O, Brooks DJ, Melamed E, Oertel W, Poewe W, Stocchi F, Tolosa E; LARGO study group. Rasagiline as an adjunct to levodopa in patients with Parkinson's disease and motor fluctuations (LARGO, Lasting effect in Adjunct therapy with Rasagiline Given Once daily, study): a randomised, double-blind, parallel-group trial. Lancet. 2005 Mar 12-18;365(9463): 914-6.

106. Parkinson Study Group. A randomized placebo-controlled trial of rasagiline in levodopa-treated patients with Parkinson disease and motor fluctuations: the PRESTO study. Arch Neurol. 2005 Feb;62(2):241-8.

107. Parkinson Study Group. A controlled trial of rasagiline in early Parkinson's disease. The TEMPO study. Arch neruol 2002;59:1937-1943.

108. Rascol O, Brooks DJ, Melamed E, Oertel W, Poewe W, Stocchi F, Tolosa E; LARGO study group. Rasagiline as an adjunct to levodopa in patients with Parkinson's disease and motor fluctuations (LARGO, Lasting effect in Adjunct therapy with Rasagiline Given Once daily, study): a randomised, double-blind, parallel-group trial. Lancet. 2005 Mar 12-18;365(9463): 914-6.

109. Jabbari B, Scherokman B, Gunderson CH et al. Treatment of movement disorders with trihexyphenidyl. Mov Disord 1989;4:202-212.

110. Butzer JF, Silver DE, Sahs AL. Amantadine in Parkinson's disease: a double-blind placebo-controlled cross-over study with long-term follow-up. Neurology 1975;25:603-606.

111. Metman LV, DelDotto P, van DenMunckhof P et al. Amantadine as treatment for dyskinesias and motor fluctuations in Parkinson's disease. Neurology 1998;50:1323-1326.

112. Metman LV, DelDotto P, LePoole K et al. Amantadine for levodopa-induced dyskinesias. A one-year follow-up study. Arch Neurol 1999;56:1383-1386.

113. Gerlak RP, Clark R, Stump JM et al. Amantadine-dopamine interaction. Science 1970;169:203-204.

114. Rajput AH, levodopa prolongs life expectancy and is non-toxic to substantia nigra Parkinsonism Relat Disord 2001;8:95-100.

115. Parkinson Study Group. Levodopa and the progression of Parkison's disease. N Engl J Med. 2004 dec 9;351(24):2498-508.

Chapter 7

1. Parkinson Study Group. A controlled trial of rasagiline in early Parkinson disease: the TEMPO Study. Arch Neurol. 2002 Dec;59(12):1937-43.

2. Pearce RK, Banerji T, Jenner P, Marsden CD. De novo administration of ropinirole and bromocriptine induces less dyskinesia than levodopa in MPTP-treated marmosets. Mov Disord 1998;13:234-241.

3. Montastruc JL, Rascol O, Senard JM, Rascol A. A randomised controlled study comparing bromocriptine to which levodopa was later added, with levodopa alone in previously untreated patients with Parkinson's disease: a five-year follow up. J Neurol Neurosurg Psychiatry 1994;57:1034-1038.

4. Parkinson Study Group. Pramipexole vs levodopa as initial treatment for Parkinson disease: A randomized controlled trial. JAMA 2000;284:1931-8.

5. Rascol O, Brooks DJ, Korczyn AD, De Deyn PP, Clarke CE, Lang AE. A five-year study of the incidence of dyskinesia in patients with early Parkinson's disease who were treated with ropinirole or levodopa. 056 Study Group. N Engl J Med 2000;342:1484-91.

6. Metman LV, DelDotto P, van DenMunckhof P et al. Amantadine as treatment for dyskinesia and motor fluctuations in Parkinson's disease. Neurology 1998;50:1323-1326.

7. Pereira da Silva-Junior F, Braga-Neto P, Sueli Monte F, Meireles Sales de Bruin V. Amantadine reduces the duration of levodopa-induced dyskinesia: a randomized, double-blind, placebo-controlled study. Parkinsonism Relat Disord 2005;11:449-52.

8. Dewey RB Jr, Hutton JT, LeWitt PA, Factor SA. A randomized, double-blind, placebo-controlled trial of subcutaneously injected apomorphine for parkinsonian off-state events. Arch Neurol 2001;58:1385-92.

9. Factor SA. Literature review: intermittent subcutaneous apomorphine therapy in Parkinson's disease. Neurology 2004;62(Suppl 4):S12-7.

10. Carter JH, Nutt JG, Woodward WR, Hatcher LF, Trotman TL. Amount and distribution of dietary protein affects clinical response to levodopa in Parkinson's disease. Neurology 1989;39:552-556.

11. Kurth MC, Tetrud JW, Irwin I, Lynes WH, Langston JW. Oral levodopa/carbidopa solution versus tablets in Parkinson's disease patients with severe fluctuations: a pilot study. Neurology 1993;43:1036-1039.

12. Lieberman A, Dziatolowski M, Kupersmith M, Serby M, Goodgold A, Korein J, Goldstein M. Dementia in Parkinson's disease. Ann Neurol 1979;6:355-359.

13. Baldessarini RJ, Frankenburg FR. Drug therapy: clozapine-a novel antipsychotic agent. N Engl J Med 1991;324:746-756.

14. Menza MM, Palermo B, Mark M. Quetiapine as an alternativde to clozapine in the treatment of dopamimetic psychosis in patients with Parkinson's disease. Ann Clin Psychiatry 1999;11:141-144.

15. Fernandez HH, Friedman JH, Jacques C, Rosenfield M. Quetiapine for the treatment of drug-induced psychosis in Parkinson's disease. Mov Disord 1999;14:484-487.

Chapter 8

1. Gulati A, Forbes A, Stegie F, et al. A clinical observational study of the pattern and occurrence of non-motor symptoms in Parkinson's disease ranging from early to advanced disease. Mov Disord 2004;19(suppl 9):S406

2. Karlsen KH, Larsen JP, Tandberg E, et al. Influence of clinical and demographic variables on quality of life in patients with Parkinson's disease. J Neurol Neurosurg Psychiatry 1999;66:431-435.

3. Arsland D, Larsen JP, Tandberg E, Laake K. Predictors of nursing home placement in Parkinson's disease: a population based, prospective study. J Am Geriatr Soc 2000;48:938-942.

4. Findley L, Aujla MA, Bain PG, et al. Direct economic impact of Parkinson's disease: a research survey in the United Kingdom. Mov Disord 2003;18:1139-1155.

5. Shulman LM, Taback RL, Rabinstein AA, Weiner WJ. Non-recognition of depression and other non-motor symptoms in Parkinson's disease. Parkinsonism Relat Disord 2002;8:193-197.

6. Chaudhuri KR, Martinez-Martin P, Schapira AHV et al. An international multicentre pilot study of the first comprehensive self-completed non-motor symptoms questionnaire for Parkinson's disease: The NMSQuest study. Mov Disord In Press

7. Chaudhuri K R, Martinez-Martin P, Schapira A.H.V., Ondo W, Sethi K. Memebers of the PD NMS Scale Development Group.An international multicentre study validation the first screening questionnaire (NMS–quest) for competitive assessment of non motor symptoms of Parkinson's disease. Movement Disorders.2005; 20 (10): 50. 9th International Movement Disorders Congress, New Orleans, March 2005.

8. Homan CN, Wenzyl K, Suppan M, et al. Sleep attacks after acute administration of apomorphine. Mov Disord 2000;15(Suppl 3)108.

9. Arnulf I, Bonnett AM, Damier P, et al. Hallucinations, REM sleep, and Parkinson's disease. Neurology 2000;55:281-288.

10. Hobson DE, Lang AE, Martin WR, et al. Excessive daytime sleepiness and sudden-onset sleep in Parkinson's disease. A survey by the Canadian Movement Disorders Group. JAMA 2002;287:455-463.

11. Lee MS, Rinne JO, Marsden CD. The pedunculopontine nucleus: its role in the genesis of movement disorders.Yonsei Med J 2000;41:167-184.

12. ndo WG, Dat Vuon G, Khan H, et al. Daytime sleepiness and other sleep disorders in Parkinson's disease. Neurology 2001;57:1392-1396.

13. Etminan M, Samii A, Takkouche B, Rochon PA. Increased risk of somnolence with the new dopamine agonists in patients with Parkinson's disease: a meta-analysis of randomized controlled trials. Drug Saf 2001;24(11):863-868.

14. Parkinson Study Group. Pramipexole vs levodopa as initial treatment for Parkinson's disease. A randomized controlled trial. JAMA 2000;284:1931-1938.

15. Tandberg E, Larsen JP, Karlsen K. A community-based study of sleep disorders in patients with Parkinson's disease. Mov Disord 1998;13:895-899.

16. Factor SA, McAlarney T, Sanchez-Ramos JR, Weiner WJ. Sleep disorders and sleep effect in Parkinson's disease. Mov Disord. 1990;5(4):280-5. Related Articles, Links

17. Caap-Ahlgren M, Dehlin O. Insomnia and depressive symptoms in patients with Parkinson's disease. Relationship to health-related quality of life. An interview study of patients living at home. Arch Gerontol Geriatr. 2001 Feb;32(1):23-33. Related Articles, Links

18. Arnulf I, Konofal E, Merino-Andreu M, et al. Parkinson's disease and sleepiness: an integral part of PD. Neurology 2002;58:1019-1024.

19. Beove BF, Silber MH, Ferman TJ, et al. Association of REM sleep behavior disorder and neurodegenerative disease may reflect an underlying synucleinopathy. Mov Disord 2001; 16:622-630.

20. Adler CH, Thorpy MJ. Sleep issues in Parkinson's disease. Neurology 2005;64(Suppl 3):S12-S20.

21. Comella CL, Tanner CM, Ristanovic RK. Polysomnographic sleep measures in Parkinson's disease patients with treatment-induced hallucinations. Ann Neurol 1993; 34: 710-714.

22. Morrison AR. The pathophysiology of REM-sleep behavior disorder. Sleep 1998;21:446-449.

23. Oksenberg A, Radwan H, Arons E, et al. Rapid eye movement (REM) sleep behavior disorder: a sleep disturbance affecting mainly older men. Isr J Psychiatry Relat Sci 2002;39:28-35.

24. Hogl B, Saletu M, Brandauer E, et al.Modafinil for the treatment of daytime sleepiness in Parkinson's disease: a double-blind, randomized, crossover, placebo-controlled polygraphic trial. Sleep 2002 Dec;25(8):905-9.

25. Adler CH, Caviness JN, Hentz JG, et al. Randomized trial of modafinil for treating subjective daytime sleepiness in patients with Parkinson's disease. Mov Disord. 2003 Mar;18(3):287-93.

26. Arnulf I. Excessive daytime sleepiness in parkinsonism. Sleep Med Rev. 2005 Jun;9(3):185-200. Epub 2005 Apr 26.

27. Brodsky MA, Godbold J, Olanow CW. Sleepiness in Parkinson's diseasea. Parkinsonism Relat Disord 2001;7:S93.

28. Frucht S, Roger JD, Green PE, et al. Falling asleep at the wheel: motor vehicle mishaps in persons taking pramipexole and ropinirole. Neurology 1999;52:19080-1910.

29. Olanow CW, Schapria AH, Roth T. Waking up to sleep episodes in Parkinson's disease. Mov Disord 2000;15(2):212-215.

30. Pappert EJ, Goetz CG, Niederman FG, et al. Hallucinations, sleep fragmentation, and altered dream phenomena in Parkinson's disease. Mov Disord. 1999 Jan;14(1):117-21

31. Friedman JH, Friedman H. Fatigue in Parkinson's disease: a nine-year follow-up. Mov Disord. 2001 Nov;16(6):1120-2. Related Articles, Links

32. Friedman J, Friedman H. Fatigue in Parkinson's disease. Neurology. 1993 Oct;43(10):2016-8.

33. Brown RG, Dittner A, Findley L, Wessely SC. The Parkinson fatigue scale. Parkinsonism Relat Disord. 2005 Jan;11(1):49-55

34. Awerbuch GI, Sandyk R. Autonomic functions in the early stages of Parkinson's disease. Int J Neurosci. 1992 May-Jun;64(1-4):7-14.

35. Wang SJ, Fuh JL, Shan DE, et al. Sympathetic skin response and R-R interval variation in Parkinson's disease. Mov Disord. 1993 Apr;8(2):151-7.

36. Kremer HP. The hypothalamic lateral tuberal nucleus: normal anatomy and changes in neurological diseases. Prog Brain Res. 1992;93:249-61.

37. Hickler RB, Thompson GR, Fox LM, Hamlin JT. Successful treatment of orthostatic hypotension with 9-alpha-fluoronydrocortisone. N Engl J Med 1959;261:788-791.

38. Kaufman H, Brannan T, Krakoff L, Yahr MD, Mandeli J. Treatment of orthostatic hypotension due to autonomic failure with a peripheral alpha-adrenergic agonist (midodrine). Neurology 1988;38:951-956.

39. Davies B, Bannister R, Sever P. Pressor amines and monoamineoxidase inhibitors for treatment of postural hypotension in autonomic failure: limitations and hazards. Lancet 1978;1:172-175.

40. McTavish D, Goa KL. Midodrine: a review of its pharmacological properties and therapeutic use in orthostatic hypotension and secondary hypotensive disorders. Drugs 1989;38:757-777.

41. Pittner H, Stormann H, Enzenhofer R. Pharmacodynamic actions of midodrine, a new alpha-adrenergic stimulating agent, and its main metabolite, ST 1059. Arzneim Forsch 1976; 26:2145-2154.

42. Zachariah PK, Bloedow DC, Moyer TP, Sheps SG, Schirger A, et al. Pharmacodynamics of midodrine, an antihypotensive agent. Clin Pharmacol Ther 1986;39:586-591.

43. Jankovic J, Gilden JL, Hiner BC, Kaufman H, Brown DC. Neurogenic orthostatic hypotension: a double-blind placebo-controlled study with midodrine. Am J Med 1993;95:38-48.

44. Jost WH, Schimrigk K. Constipation in Parkinson's disease. Klinische Wochenschrift 1991; 69:906-909.

45. Edwards LL, Quigley EMM, Harned RK, Hofman R, Pfeiffer R. Characterization of swallowing and defecation in Parkinson's disease. Am J Gastroenterol 1994;89:15-25.

46. Ashraf W, Pfeiffer R, Quigely EMM. Anorectal manometer in the assessment of anorectal function in Parkinson's disease: a comparison with chronic idiopathic constipation. Mov Disord 1994;9:655-663.

47. Mathers SE, Kempster PA, Law PJ, et al. Anal sphincter dysfunction in Parkinson's disease. Arch Neurol 1989;46:1061-1064.

48. Oyanagi K, Wakabayashi K, Ohama E, Takeda S, Horikawa Y, Morita T, Ikuta F. Lewy bodies in the lower sacral parasympathetic neurons of a patient with Parkinson's disease. Acta Neuropathol 1990;80:558-559.

49. Mathers SE, Kempster PA, Swash M, Lees AJ. Constipation and paradoxical puborectalis contraction in anismus and Parkinson's disease: a dystonic phenomenon? J Neurol Neurosurg Psych 1988;51:1503-1507.

50. Sullivan KL, Staffetti JF, Hauser RA, et al. Tegaserod (Zelnorm) for the treatment of constipation in Parkinson's disease. Mov Disord. 2005 Sep 2.

51. Liu Z, Sakakibara R, Odaka T, Uchiyama T,et al. Mosapride citrate, a novel 5-HT4 agonist and partial 5-HT3 antagonist, ameliorates constipation in parkinsonian patients. Mov Disord. 2005 Jun;20(6):680-6.

52. Bird MR, Woodward MC, Gibson EM, Phyland DJ, Fonda D. Asymptomatic swallowing disorders in elderly patients with Parkinson's disease: a description of findings on clinical examination and videofluoroscopy in sixteen patients. Age and Ageing 1994;23:251-254.

53. Qualman SJ, Haupt HM, Yang P, Hamilton SR. Esophageal Lewy bodies associated with ganglion cell loss in achalasia. Similarity to Parkinson's disease. Gastroenterology 1984;87:848-856.

54. Wang SJ, Chia LG, Hsu CY, Lin WY, Kao CH, Yeh SH. Dysphagia in Parkinson's disease. Assessment by solid phase radionuclide scintigraphy. Clin Nuc Med 1994;19:405-407.

55. Wintzen AR, Badrising UA, Roos RA, Vielvoye J, Liauw L, Pauwels EK. Dysphagia in ambulant patients with Parkinson's disease: common, not dangerous. Can J Neur Sci 1994;212:53-56.

56. Bushman M, Dobmeyer SM, Leeker L, Perlmutter JS. Swallowing abnormalities and their responses to treatment in Parkinson's disease. Neurology 1989;39:1309-1314.

57. Khan Z, Starer P, Bhola A. Urinary incontinence in female Parkinson's disease patients. Urology 1989;33:486-489.

58. Suchowersky O, Furtado S, Rohs G. Beneficial effect of intranasal desmopressin for nocturnal polyuria in Parkinson's disease. Mov Disord1995;10:337-340

59. Edwards LL, Pfeiffer RF, Quigley EMM, Hofman R, Balluff M. Gastrointestinal symptoms in Parkinson's disease. Movement Disorders 1991;6:151-156.

60. Edwards LL, Quigley EMM, Pfeiffer RF. Gastrointestinal dysfunction in Parkinson's disease: frequency and pathophysiology. Neurology 1992;42:726-732.

61. Hyson HC, Johnson AM, Jog MS. Sublingual atropine for sialorrhea secondary to parkinsonism: a pilot study. Mov Disord. 2002 Nov;17(6):1318-20. Related Articles, Links

62. Muller T. Drug treatment of non-motor symptoms in Parkinson's disease. Expert Opin Pharmacother. 2002 Apr;3(4):381-8. Related Articles, Links

63. Lipe, H, Longstreth WT, Bird TD, Linde M. Sexual function in married men with Parkinson's disease compared to married men with arthritis. Neurology 1990;40:1347-1349.

64. Rosen RC, Kostis JB, Jekelis AW. Beta-blocker effects on sexual function in normal males. Arch Sex Behavior 1988;17:241-55.

65. Smith PJ, Talbert RL. Sexual dysfunction with antihypertensive and antipsychotic agents. Clinical Pharmacy 1986;5:373-84.

66. Zesiewicz TA, Helal M, Hauser RA. Sildenafil Citrate (Viagra) for the treatment of erectile dysfunction in men with Parkinson's disease. Mov Disord 2000;15:305-308.

67. Cummings JL. Depression and Parkinson's disease: a review. Am J Psychiatry 1992;149:443-454.

68. Ehmann TS, Beninger RJ, Gawal MJ, Riopelle RJ. Depressive symptoms in Parkinson's disease: a comparison with disabled control subjects. J Geriatr Psychiatry Neurol 1990;2:3-9.

69. Starkstein SE, Preziosi TJ, Bolduc PL, Robinson RG. Depression in Parkinson's disease. J Nerv Ment Dis 1990;178:27-31.

70. Gotham AM, Brown RG, Marsden CD. Depression in Parkinson's disease: a quantitative and qualitative analysis. J Neurol Neurosurg Psychiatry 1986;49:381-389.

71. Celesia GC, Wanamaker WM. Psychiatric disturbances in Parkinson's disease. Dis Nerv Syst 1972;33:577-583.

72. Mayeux R, Stern Y, Williams JBW, Cote L, Frantz A, Dyrenfurth I. Clinical and biochemical features of depression in Parkinson's disease. Am J Psychiatry 1986;143:756-759.

73. Beck AT. Depression: Causes and Treatment. University of Pennsylvania Press, 1967, Philadelphia, PA, pp 333-335.

74. Hedlung and Vleweg. The Hamilton Rating Scale for depression. Journal of Operational Psychiatry 1970;10(2):149-165.

75. Mayeux R, Stern Y, Sano M, Williams JB, Cote LJ. The relationship of serotonin to depression in Parkinson's disease. Mov Disord 1988;3:237-244.

76. Andersen J, Aabro E, Gulmann N, Hjelmsted A, Pedersen HE. Anti-depressive treatment in Parkinson's disease: a controlled trial of the effect of nortriptyline in patients with Parkinson's disease treated with L-dopa. Acta Neurol Scan 1980;52:210-219.

77. Laitenen L. Desipramine in treatment of Parkinson's disease. Acta Neurol Scand 1969;45: 109-113.

78. Goetz CG, Tanner CM, Klawans HL. Bupropion in Parkinson's disease. Neurology 1984;34:1092-1094.

79. Jansen-Steur ENH. Increase of Parkinson disability after fluoxetine medication. Neurology 1993;43:211-213.

80. Jiménez-Jimenez FJ, Tejeiro J, Martinez-Junquera G, Cabrera-Valdivia F, Alarcon J, et al. Parkinsonism exacerbated by paroxetine. Neurology 1994;44:2406.

81. Hauser RA, Zesiewicz TA. Sertraline for the treatment of depression in Parkinson's disease. Mov Disord 1997;12:756-759.

82. Sternbach H. The serotonin syndrome. Am J Psychiatry 1991;148:705-713.

83. Nirenberg DW, Semprebon M. The central nervous system serotonin syndrome. Clin Pharmacol Ther 1993;84-88.

84. Tackley RM, Tregaskis B. Fatal disseminated intravascular coagulation following a monoamine oxidase inhibitor/tricyclic interaction. Anaesthesia 1987;42:760-763.

85. Corkeron MA. Serotonin syndrome - a potentially fatal complication of antidepressant therapy. Med J Austral 1995;163:481-482.

86. Waters CH. Fluoxetine and selegiline - lack of significant interaction. Can J Neurol 1994; 21:259-261.

87. Richard IH, Kurlan R, Tanner C et al. Serotonin syndrome and the combined use of deprenyl and an antidepressant in Parkinson's disease. Parkinson Study Group. Neurology 1997;48:1070-1077.

88. Richard IH. Anxiety disorders in Parkinson's disease. Adv Neurol. 2005;96:42-55. Links

89. Witjas T, Kaphan E, Azulay JP, et al. Nonmotor fluctuations in Parkinson's disease: frequent and disabling. Neurology2002;59:408-413.

90. Emre M. Dementia associated with Parkinson's disease. Lancet Neurol. 2003;2(4):229-237.

91. Aarsland D, Andersen K, Larsen J, et al. Prevalence and characteristics of dementia in Parkinson's disease: an 8-year prospective study. Arch Neurol 2003;60:387-392.

92. Peran P, Rascol O, Demonet JF, et al. Deficit of verb generation in non-demented patients with Parkinson's disease. Mov Disord 2003;18:150-156.

93. Agid Y, Ruberg M, Dubois B et al. Parkinson's disease and dementia. Clin Neuropharm 1986;9:S22-36.

94. Parashos SA, Maraganore DM, O'Brien PC, Rocca WA. Medical services utilization and prognosis in Parkinson disease: a population-based study. Mayo Clin Proc. 2002 Sep;77(9):918-25.

95. Hurtig HI, Trojanowski JQ, Galvin J, et al. Alpha-synuclein cortical Lewy bodies correlate with dementia in Parkinson's disease. Neurology. 2000 May 23;54(10):1916-21.

96. Ravina B, Putt M, Siderowf A, et al. Donopezil for dementia in Parkinson's disease: a randomized, double-blind, placebo controlled, crossover study. J Neurol Neurosurg Psychiatry 2005;76(7):934-939.

97. Emre M, Aarsland D, Albanese A, et al. Rivastigmine for dementia associated with Parkinson's disease. N Engl J Med 2004;351(24):2509-2518.

98. Naimark D, Jackson E, Rockwell E, Jeste DV. Psychotic symptoms in Parkinson's disease patients with dementia. J Am Geriatr Soc. 1996 Mar;44(3):296-9.

99. Thanvi BR, Lo TC, Harsh DP. Psychosis in Parkinson's disease. Postgrad Med J. 2005 Oct;81(960):644-646.

100. Sanchez-Ramos JR, Ortoll R, Paulson GW. Visual hallucinations associated with Parkinson disease. Arch Neurol. 1996 Dec;53(12):1265-8.

Chapter 9

1. Soykan I, Sarosiek I, Shifflett J, Wooten GF, McCallum RW. Effect of chronic oral domperidone therapy on gastrointestinal symptoms and gastric emptying in patients with Parkinson's disease. Mov Disord 1997;12:952-957.

2. Poewe WH, Lees AJ, Stern GM. Treatment of Motor Fluctuations in Parkinson's Disease with an oral Sustained-Release Preparation of L-Dopa: Clinical and Pharmacokinetic Observations. Clin. Neuropharm 1986; 9: 430-439.

3. UK Madopar CR Study Group. A comparison of Madopar CR and Standard Madopar in the treatment of nocturnal and early-morning disability in Parkinson's disease. Clin Neuropharmacol 1989;12:498-505

4. Descombes S, Bonnet AM, Gasser UE et al. Dual-release formulation, a novel principle in L-Dopa treatment of Parkinson's disease. Neurology 2001;56:1239-1242.

5. Contin M, Riva R, Martinelli P, Cortelli P, Albani F, Baruzzi A. Concentration-effect relationship of levodopa-benserazide formulation versus standard formulation in the treatment of complicated motor response fluctuations in Parkinson's disease. Clin Neuropharmacol 1999;22:351-355.

6. Quinn N, Parkes JD, Marsden CD. Control of on/off phenomenon by continuous intravenous infusion of levodopa. Neurology, 1984;34:1131-1136.

7. Hardie RJ, Less AJ, Stern GM . On-off fluctuations in Parkinson's disease. A clinical and neuropharmacological study. Brain 1984;107:487-506.

8. Nutt JG, Fellman JH. Pharmacokinetics of levodopa. Clin Neuropharmacol 1984;7:35-49.

9. Kurth MC, Tetrud JW, Tanner CM et al . Double-blind, Placebo controlled, cross over study of duodenal infusion of levodopa/carbidopa in Parkinson's disease patient with On-Off fluctuations. Neurology 1993;43:1698-1703.

10. Syed N, Murphey J, Zimmerman T Jr, Mark MH, Sage JI . Ten year's experience with enteral levodopa infusion for motor fluctuations in Parkinson's disease. Mov Disord 1998;13:336-338.

11. Nyholm D, Nilsson Remahl A, Dizdar N et al. Duodenal levodopa infusion monotherapy versus oral pharmacy in advanced Parkinson's disease. Neurology 2005;64:216-223.

12. Mourandin MM, Heuser IJ, Baronti F, Chase TN . Modification of central dopaminergic mechanisms by continuous levodopa therapy for advanced parkinson's disease. Ann Neurol 1990;27:18-23.

13. Nyholm D, Aquilonius SM. . Levodopa infusion therapy in Parkinson's disease: State of the Art in 2004. Clin Neuropharmacol 2004;27:245-256.

14. Rinne UK, Bracco F, Chouza C et al. Cabergoline in the treatment of early Parkinson's disease: results of the first year of treatment in a double-blind, comparison of cabergoline and levodopa. Neurology 1997;48:363-368.

15. Rinne UK, Braco F, Chouza C et al. Early treatment of Parkinson's disease with Cabergoline delays the onset of motor complications. Drugs 1998;5(suppl):23-30.

16. Inzelberg R, Nisipeanu P, Rabey JM et al. Double-blind comparison of Cabergoline and Bromocriptine in Parkinson's disease patients with motor fluctuations. Neurology 1996;47:785-788.

17. Hutton JT, Koller WC, Ahlskog JE et al. Multicenter, placebo-controlled trial of Cabergoline taken once daily in the treatment of Parkinson's disease. Neurology 1996;46:1062-1065.

18. Horvath J, Fross RD, Kleiner Fishman G et al. Severe multivalvular heart disease: a new complication of the ergot derivative dopamine agonists. Mov Disord 2004;19:656-562.

19. Pinero A, Marcos-Alberca P, Fortes J . Cabergoline-related severe restrictive mitral regurgitation. N Engl J Med 2005; 353:1976-1977.

20. Peralta C, Wolf E, Alber H et al. Valvular heart disease in Parkinson's Disease vs controls: An echocardiographic study. Mov Disord. In press.

21. Bergamasco B, Frattola L, Muratrio A, Piccoli F, Mailland F, Parnetti L. Alpha-dihydroergocriptine in the treatment of de-novo parkinsonian patients: results of a multi-center, randomized, double-blind, placebo-controlled study. Acta Neurol Scand 2000; 101:372-380.

22. Albanese A, Colosimo C. . Dihydroergocriptine in Parkinson's disease: clinical efficacy and comparison with other dopamine agonists. Acta Neurol Scand 2003;107:349-355.

23. Rondot P, Ziegler M . Activity and acceptability of piribedil in Parkinson's disease: a multi-center study. J Neurol 1992;239:28-34.

24. Ziegler M, Castro-Caldas A, Del Signore S, Rascol O. Efficacy of Piribedil as early combination to levodopa in patients with stable Parkinson's disease: A 6 Month, Randomized, Placebo-controlled study. Mov Disord 2003;18:418-425.

25. Stibe CM, Lees AJ, Kempster PA, Stern GM . Subcutaneous apomorphine in parkinsonian on-off oscillations. Lancet 1988;20:403-406.

26. Hughes AJ, Bishop S, Kleedorfer B et al. Subcutaneous apomorphine in Parkinson's disease: response to chronic administration for up to five years. Mov Disord 1993;8:165-70.

27. Poewe W, Wenning GK. Apomorphine: an underutilized therapy for Parkinson's disease. Mov Disord 2000;15:789-94.

28. Colzi A, Turner K, Lees AJ. Continuous subcutaneous waking day apomorphine in the long-term treatment of levodopa induced dyskinesias in Parkinson's disease. J Neurol Neurosurg Psychiatry 1998;64:573-576.

29. Pietz K, Hagell P, Odin P . Subcutaneous apomorphine in late stage Parkinson's disease: a long-term follow up. J Neurol Neurosurg Psychiatry 1998;65:709-716.

30. Hughes AJ . Apomorphine test in the assessment of parkinsonian patients: A meta-analysis. Adv Neurol 1999;80:363-368.

31. Pinter MM, Alesch F, Murg M, Helscher RJ, Binder H . Apomorphine test: a predictor for motor responsiveness to deep brain stimulation of the subthalamic nucleus. J Neurol 1999; 246:907-913.

Chapter 10

1. Koller WC, Pahwa R, Lyons KE, Albanese A. Surgical treatment of Parkinson's disease. Journal of the Neurological Sciences. 1999;167(1):1-10.

2. Lyons KE, Pahwa R. Deep brain stimulation in Parkinson's disease. Curr Neurol Neurosci Rep 2004;4 (4):290-295.

3. Krack P, Fraix V, Mendes A, Benabid AL, Pollak P. Postoperative management of subthalamic nucleus stimulation for Parkinson's disease. Movement Disorders. 2002;17 (Suppl 3):S188-197.

4. Spiegel EA, Wycis HT. Thalamotomy and pallidotomy for treatment of choreic movements. Acta Neurochir (Wien) 1952;2(3-4):417-422.

5. Starr PA, Christine CW, Theodosopoulos PV, Lindsey N, Byrd D, Mosley A, et al. Implantation of deep brain stimulators into the subthalamic nucleus: technical approach and magnetic resonance imaging-verified lead locations. Journal of Neurosurgery. 2002;97(2):370-387.

6. Hassler R, Riechert T. [Indications and localization of stereotactic brain operations.]. Nervenarzt 1954;25(11):441-447.

7. Svennilson E, Torvik A, Lowe R, Leksell L. Treatment of parkinsonism by stereotatic thermolesions in the pallidal region. A clinical evaluation of 81 cases. Acta Psychiatr Scand 1960;35:358-377.

8. Wichmann T, Vitek JL. Physiology of the basal ganglia and pathophysiology of movement disorders. In Tarsy D, Vitek JL, Lozano AM (eds). Surgical Treatment of Parkinson's Disease and Other Movement Disorders. 2003;New Jersey: Humana Press:3-18.

9. Bakay RA, Starr PA, Vitek JL, DeLong MR. Posterior ventral pallidotomy: techniques and theoretical considerations. Clin Neurosurg 1997;44:197-210.

10. Holloway KL, Gaede SE, Starr PA, Rosenow JM, Ramakrishnan V, Henderson JM. Frameless stereotaxy using bone fiducial markers for deep brain stimulation. J Neurosurg 2005;103(3):404-413.

11. Kelly PJ, Gillingham FJ. The long-term results of stereotaxic surgery and L-dopa therapy in patients with Parkinson's disease. A 10-year follow-up study. J Neurosurg 1980;53(3):332-337.

12. Nagaseki Y, Shibazaki T, Hirai T, Kawashima Y, Hirato M, Wada H, et al. Long-term follow-up results of selective VIM-thalamotomy. J Neurosurg 1986;65(3):296-302.

13. Jankovic J, Cardoso F, Grossman RG, Hamilton WJ. Outcome after stereotactic thalamotomy for parkinsonian, essential, and other types of tremor. Neurosurgery 1995;37(4):680-686; discussion 686-687.

14. Diederich N, Goetz CG, Stebbins GT, Klawans HL, Nittner K, Koulosakis A, et al. Blinded evaluation confirms long-term asymmetric effect of unilateral thalamotomy or subthalamotomy on tremor in Parkinson's disease. Neurology 1992;42(7):1311-1314.

15. Alkhani A, Lozano AM. Pallidotomy for parkinson disease: a review of contemporary literature. J Neurosurg 2001;94(1):43-49.

16. Lang AE, Lozano AM, Montgomery E, Duff J, Tasker R, Hutchinson W. Posteroventral medial pallidotomy in advanced Parkinson's disease. N Engl J Med 1997;337(15):1036-1042.

17. Pal PK, Samii A, Kishore A, Schulzer M, Mak E, Yardley S, et al. long-term outcome of unilateral pallidotomy: follow up of 15 patients for 3 years. J Neurol Neurosurg Psychiatry 2000;69(3):337-344.

18. Hariz MI, Bergenheim AT. A 10-year follow-up review of patients who underwent Leksell's posteroventral pallidotomy for Parkinson disease. J Neurosurg 2001;94(4):552-558.

19. Alvarez L, Macias R, Lopez G, Alvarez E, Pavon N, Rodriguez-Oroz MC, et al. Bilateral subthalamotomy in Parkinson's disease: initial and long-term response. Brain 2005;128(Pt 3):570-583.

20. Alvarez L, Macias R, Guridi J, Lopez G, Alvarez E, Maragoto C, et al. Dorsal subthalamotomy for Parkinson's disease. Mov Disord 2001;16(1):72-78.

21. de Bie RM, de Haan RJ, Schuurman PR, Esselink RA, Bosch DA, Speelman JD. Morbidity and mortality following pallidotomy in Parkinson's disease: a systematic review. Neurology 2002;58(7):1008-1012.

22. De Bie RM, Schuurman PR, Esselink RA, Bosch DA, Speelman JD. Bilateral pallidotomy in Parkinson's disease: a retrospective study. Mov Disord 2002;17(3):533-538.

23. Intemann PM, Masterman D, Subramanian I, DeSalles A, Behnke E, Frysinger R, et al. Staged bilateral pallidotomy for treatment of Parkinson disease. J Neurosurg 2001;94(3):437-444.

24. Benabid AL, Pollak P, Louveau A, Henry S, de Rougemont J. Combined (thalamotomy and stimulation) stereotactic surgery of the VIM thalamic nucleus for bilateral Parkinson disease. Applied Neurophysiology. 1987;50(1-6):344-346.

25. Lozano AM, Eltahawy H. How does DBS work? Suppl Clin Neurophysiol 2004;57:733-736.

26. Pollak P, Benabid AL, Limousin P, Benazzouz A. Chronic intracerebral stimulation in Parkinson's disease. Advances in Neurology. 1997;74:213-220.

27. Blond S, Siegfried J. Thalamic stimulation for the treatment of tremor and other movement disorders. Acta Neurochirurgica - Supplementum. 1991;52:109-111.

28. Alesch F, Pinter MM, Helscher RJ, Fertl L, Benabid AL, Koos WT. Stimulation of the ventral intermediate thalamic nucleus in tremor dominated Parkinson's disease and essential tremor. Acta Neurochirurgica. 1995;136(1-2):75-81.

29. Benabid AL, Pollak P, Gao D, Hoffmann D, Limousin P, Gay E, et al. Chronic electrical stimulation of the ventralis intermedius nucleus of the thalamus as a treatment of movement disorders.[comment]. Journal of Neurosurgery. 1996;84(2):203-214.

30. Koller W, Pahwa R, Busenbark K, Hubble J, Wilkinson S, Lang A, et al. High-frequency unilateral thalamic stimulation in the treatment of essential and parkinsonian tremor. Annals of Neurology. 1997;42(3):292-299.

31. Limousin P, Speelman JD, Gielen F, Janssens M. Multicentre European study of thalamic stimulation in parkinsonian and essential tremor. Journal of Neurology, Neurosurgery & Psychiatry. 1999;66(3):289-296.

32. Ondo W, Jankovic J, Schwartz K, Almaguer M, Simpson RK. Unilateral thalamic deep brain stimulation for refractory essential tremor and Parkinson's disease tremor. Neurology. 1998;51(4):1063-1069.

33. Lyons KE, Koller WC, Wilkinson SB, Pahwa R. long-term safety and efficacy of unilateral deep brain stimulation of the thalamus for parkinsonian tremor. Journal of Neurology, Neurosurgery & Psychiatry. 2001;71(5):682-684.

34. Rehncrona S, Johnels B, Widner H, Tornqvist AL, Hariz M, Sydow O. Long-term efficacy of thalamic deep brain stimulation for tremor: double-blind assessments. Movement Disorders. 2003;18(2):163-170.

35. Kumar R, Lozano AM, Montgomery E, Lang AE. Pallidotomy and deep brain stimulation of the pallidum and subthalamic nucleus in advanced Parkinson's disease. Movement Disorders. 1998;13(Suppl 1):73-82.

36. Kumar R, Lang AE, Rodriguez-Oroz MC, Lozano AM, Limousin P, Pollak P, et al. Deep brain stimulation of the globus pallidus pars interna in advanced Parkinson's disease. Neurology. 2000;55(12 Suppl 6):S34-39.

37. The Deep-Brain Stimulation for Parkinson's Disease Study G. Deep-brain stimulation of the subthalamic nucleus or the pars interna of the globus pallidus in Parkinson's disease.[comment]. New England Journal of Medicine. 2001;345(13):956-963.

38. Ghika J, Villemure JG, Fankhauser H, Favre J, Assal G, Ghika-Schmid F. Efficiency and safety of bilateral contemporaneous pallidal stimulation (deep brain stimulation) in levodopa-responsive patients with Parkinson's disease with severe motor fluctuations: a 2-year follow-up review. Journal of Neurosurgery. 1998;89(5):713-718.

39. Volkmann J, Sturm V, Weiss P, Kappler J, Voges J, Koulousakis A, et al. Bilateral high-frequency stimulation of the internal globus pallidus in advanced Parkinson's disease. Annals of Neurology. 1998;44(6):953-961.

40. Durif F, Lemaire JJ, Debilly B, Dordain G. Long-term follow-up of globus pallidus chronic stimulation in advanced Parkinson's disease. Movement Disorders. 2002;17(4):803-807.

41. Lyons KE, Wilkinson SB, Troster AI, Pahwa R. Long-term efficacy of globus pallidus stimulation for the treatment of Parkinson's disease. Stereotact Funct Neurosurg 2002;79(3-4):214-220.

42. Kumar R, Lozano AM, Kim YJ, Hutchison WD, Sime E, Halket E, et al. Double-blind evaluation of subthalamic nucleus deep brain stimulation in advanced Parkinson's disease. Neurology. 1998;51(3):850-855.

43. Limousin P, Krack P, Pollak P, Benazzouz A, Ardouin C, Hoffmann D, et al. Electrical stimulation of the subthalamic nucleus in advanced Parkinson's disease. New England Journal of Medicine. 1998;339(16):1105-1111.

44. Krack P, Pollak P, Limousin P, Hoffmann D, Xie J, Benazzouz A, et al. Subthalamic nucleus or internal pallidal stimulation in young onset Parkinson's disease. Brain. 1998;121(Pt 3):451-457.

45. Benabid AL, Krack PP, Benazzouz A, Limousin P, Koudsie A, Pollak P. Deep brain stimulation of the subthalamic nucleus for Parkinson's disease: methodologic aspects and clinical criteria. Neurology. 2000;55(12 Suppl 6):S40-44.

46. Rodriguez-Oroz MC, Gorospe A, Guridi J, Ramos E, Linazasoro G, Rodriguez-Palmero M, et al. Bilateral deep brain stimulation of the subthalamic nucleus in Parkinson's disease. Neurology. 2000;55(12 Suppl 6):S45-51.

47. Romito LM, Scerrati M, Contarino MF, Bentivoglio AR, Tonali P, Albanese A. Long-term follow up of subthalamic nucleus stimulation in Parkinson's disease. Neurology. 2002;58(10):1546-1550.

48. Pahwa R, Wilkinson SB, Overman J, Lyons KE. Bilateral subthalamic stimulation in patients with Parkinson disease: long-term follow up. Journal of Neurosurgery. 2003;99(1):71-77.

49. Kleiner-Fisman G, Fisman DN, Sime E, Saint-Cyr JA, Lozano AM, Lang AE. Long-term follow up of bilateral deep brain stimulation of the subthalamic nucleus in patients with advanced Parkinson disease. Journal of Neurosurgery. 2003;99(3):489-495.

50. Krack P, Batir A, Van Blercom N, Chabardes S, Fraix V, Ardouin C, et al. Five-year follow-up of bilateral stimulation of the subthalamic nucleus in advanced Parkinson's disease.[see comment]. New England Journal of Medicine. 2003;349(20):1925-1934.

51. Burchiel KJ, Anderson VC, Favre J, Hammerstad JP. Comparison of pallidal and subthalamic nucleus deep brain stimulation for advanced Parkinson's disease: results of a randomized, blinded pilot study. Neurosurgery. 1999;45(6):1375-1382; discussion 1382-1374.

52. Volkmann J, Allert N, Voges J, Weiss PH, Freund HJ, Sturm V. Safety and efficacy of pallidal or subthalamic nucleus stimulation in advanced PD.[erratum appears in Neurology 2001 Oct 9;57(7):1354]. Neurology. 2001;56(4):548-551.

53. Scotto di Luzio A, Ammannati F, Marini P, Sorbi S, Mennonna P. Which target for DBS in Parkinson's disease? Subthalamic nucleus versus globus pallidus internus. Neurol Sci 2001;Feb;22(1):87-88.

54. Krause M, Fogel W, Heck A, Hacke W, Bonsanto M, Trenkwalder C, et al. Deep brain stimulation for the treatment of Parkinson's disease: subthalamic nucleus versus globus pallidus internus. Journal of Neurology, Neurosurgery & Psychiatry. 2001;70(4):464-470.

55. Welter ML, Houeto JL, Tezenas du Montcel S, Mesnage V, Bonnet AM, Pillon B, et al. Clinical predictive factors of subthalamic stimulation in Parkinson's disease. Brain. 2002;125(Pt 3):575-583.

56. Charles PD, Van Blercom N, Krack P, Lee SL, Xie J, Besson G, et al. Predictors of effective bilateral subthalamic nucleus stimulation for PD. Neurology. 2002;59(6):932-934.

57. Jaggi JL, Umemura A, Hurtig HI, Siderowf AD, Colcher A, Stern MB, et al. Bilateral stimulation of the subthalamic nucleus in Parkinson's disease: surgical efficacy and prediction of outcome. Stereotact Funct Neurosurg 2004;82(2-3):104-114.

58. Pahwa R, Wilkinson SB, Overman J, Lyons KE. Preoperative clinical predictors of response to bilateral subthalamic stimulation in patients with Parkinson's disease. Stereotact Funct Neurosurg 2005;83(2-3):80-83.

59. Beric A, Kelly PJ, Rezai A, Sterio D, Mogilner A, Zonenshayn M, et al. Complications of deep brain stimulation surgery.Stereotactic & Functional Neurosurgery. 2001;77(1-4):73-78.

60. Oh MY, Abosch A, Kim SH, Lang AE, Lozano AM. Long-term hardware-related complications of deep brain stimulation. Neurosurgery. 2002;50(6):1268-1274; discussion 1274-1266.

61. Umemura A, Jaggi JL, Hurtig HI, Siderowf AD, Colcher A, Stern MB, et al. Deep brain stimulation for movement disorders: morbidity and mortality in 109 patients. Journal of Neurosurgery. 2003;98(4):779-784.

62. Lyons KE, Wilkinson SB, Overman J, Pahwa R. Surgical and hardware complications of subthalamic stimulation: a series of 160 procedures. Neurology 2004;63(4):612-616.

63. Lindvall O, Backlund EO, Farde L, Sedvall G, Freedman R, Hoffer B, et al. Transplantation in Parkinson's disease: two cases of adrenal medullary grafts to the putamen. Ann Neurol 1987;22(4):457-468.

64. Backlund EO, Granberg PO, Hamberger B, Knutsson E, Martensson A, Sedvall G, et al. Transplantation of adrenal medullary tissue to striatum in parkinsonism. First clinical trials. J Neurosurg 1985;62(2):169-173.

65. Madrazo I, Drucker-Colin R, Diaz V, Martinez-Mata J, Torres C, Becerril JJ. Open microsurgical autograft of adrenal medulla to the right caudate nucleus in two patients with intractable Parkinson's disease. N Engl J Med 1987;316(14):831-834.

66. Allen GS, Burns RS, Tulipan NB, Parker RA. Adrenal medullary transplantation to the caudate nucleus in Parkinson's disease. Initial clinical results in 18 patients. Arch Neurol 1989;46(5):487-491.

67. Jankovic J, Grossman R, Goodman C, Pirozzolo F, Schneider L, Zhu Z, et al. Clinical, biochemical, and neuropathologic findings following transplantation of adrenal medulla to the caudate nucleus for treatment of Parkinson's disease. Neurology 1989;39(9):1227-1234.

68. Ahlskog JE, Kelly PJ, van Heerden JA, Stoddard SL, Tyce GM, Windebank AJ, et al. Adrenal medullary transplantation into the brain for treatment of Parkinson's disease: clinical outcome and neurochemical studies. Mayo Clin Proc 1990;65(3):305-328.

69. Olanow CW, Koller W, Goetz CG, Stebbins GT, Cahill DW, Gauger LL, et al. Autologous transplantation of adrenal medulla in Parkinson's disease. 18-month results. Arch Neurol 1990;47(12):1286-1289.

70. Goetz CG, Stebbins GT, 3rd, Klawans HL, Koller WC, Grossman RG, Bakay RA, et al. United Parkinson Foundation Neurotransplantation Registry on adrenal medullary transplants: presurgical, and 1- and 2-year follow-up. Neurology 1991;41(11):1719-1722.

71. Hurtig H, Joyce J, Sladek JR, Jr., Trojanowski JQ. Postmortem analysis of adrenal-medulla-to-caudate autograft in a patient with Parkinson's disease. Ann Neurol 1989;25(6):607-614.

72. Waters C, Itabashi HH, Apuzzo ML, Weiner LP. Adrenal to caudate transplantation--postmortem study. Mov Disord 1990;5(3):248-250.

73. Brundin P, Bjorklund A. Survival, growth and function of dopaminergic neurons grafted to the brain. Prog Brain Res 1987;71:293-308.

74. Sladek JR, Jr., Collier TJ, Haber SN, Roth RH, Redmond DE, Jr. Survival and growth of fetal catecholamine neurons transplanted into primate brain. Brain Res Bull 1986;17(6):809-818.

75. Bakay RA, Barrow DL, Fiandaca MS, Iuvone PM, Schiff A, Collins DC. Biochemical and behavioral correction of MPTP Parkinson-like syndrome by fetal cell transplantation. Ann N Y Acad Sci 1987;495:623-640.

76. Sladek JR, Jr., Redmond DE, Jr., Collier TJ, Blount JP, Elsworth JD, Taylor JR, et al. Fetal dopamine neural grafts: extended reversal of methylphenyltetrahydropyridine-induced parkinsonism in monkeys. Prog Brain Res 1988;78:497-506.

77. Fine A, Hunt SP, Oertel WH, Nomoto M, Chong PN, Bond A, et al. Transplantation of embryonic marmoset dopaminergic neurons to the corpus striatum of marmosets rendered parkinsonian by 1-methyl-4-phenyl-1,2,3,6-tetrahydropyridine. Prog Brain Res 1988;78:479-489.

78. Lindvall O, Rehncrona S, Brundin P, Gustavii B, Astedt B, Widner H, et al. Human fetal dopamine neurons grafted into the striatum in two patients with severe Parkinson's disease. A detailed account of methodology and a 6-month follow-up. Arch Neurol 1989;46(6):615-631.

79. Freed CR, Breeze RE, Rosenberg NL, Schneck SA, Kriek E, Qi JX, et al. Survival of implanted fetal dopamine cells and neurologic improvement 12 to 46 months after transplantation for Parkinson's disease. N Engl J Med 1992;327(22):1549-1555.

80. Lindvall O, Sawle G, Widner H, Rothwell JC, Bjorklund A, Brooks D, et al. Evidence for long-term survival and function of dopaminergic grafts in progressive Parkinson's disease. Ann Neurol 1994;35(2):172-180.

81. Kordower JH, Freeman TB, Snow BJ, Vingerhoets FJ, Mufson EJ, Sanberg PR, et al. Neuropathological evidence of graft survival and striatal reinnervation after the transplantation of fetal mesencephalic tissue in a patient with Parkinson's disease. N Engl J Med 1995;332(17):1118-1124.

82. Wenning GK, Odin P, Morrish P, Rehncrona S, Widner H, Brundin P, et al. Short- and long-term survival and function of unilateral intrastriatal dopaminergic grafts in Parkinson's disease. Ann Neurol 1997;42(1):95-107.

83. Kordower JH, Freeman TB, Chen EY, Mufson EJ, Sanberg PR, Hauser RA, et al. Fetal nigral grafts survive and mediate clinical benefit in a patient with Parkinson's disease. Mov Disord 1998;13(3):383-393.

84. Hauser RA, Freeman TB, Snow BJ, Nauert M, Gauger L, Kordower JH, et al. Long-term evaluation of bilateral fetal nigral transplantation in Parkinson disease. Arch Neurol 1999;56(2):179-187.

85. Piccini P, Brooks DJ, Bjorklund A, Gunn RN, Grasby PM, Rimoldi O, et al. Dopamine release from nigral transplants visualized in vivo in a Parkinson's patient. Nat Neurosci 1999;2(12):1137-1140.

86. Freed CR, Greene PE, Breeze RE, Tsai WY, DuMouchel W, Kao R, et al. Transplantation of embryonic dopamine neurons for severe Parkinson's disease. N Engl J Med 2001;344(10):710-719.

87. Olanow CW, Goetz CG, Kordower JH, Stoessl AJ, Sossi V, Brin MF, et al. A double-blind controlled trial of bilateral fetal nigral transplantation in Parkinson's disease. Ann Neurol 2003;54(3):403-414.

88. Ma Y, Feigin A, Dhawan V, Fukuda M, Shi Q, Greene P, et al. Dyskinesia after fetal cell transplantation for parkinsonism: a PET study. Ann Neurol 2002;52(5):628-634.

89. Schumacher JM, Ellias SA, Palmer EP, Kott HS, Dinsmore J, Dempsey PK, et al. Transplantation of embryonic porcine mesencephalic tissue in patients with PD. Neurology 2000;54(5):1042-1050.

90. Deacon T, Schumacher J, Dinsmore J, Thomas C, Palmer P, Kott S, et al. Histological evidence of fetal pig neural cell survival after transplantation into a patient with Parkinson's disease. Nat Med 1997;3(3):350-353.

91. Hauser RA, Watts RL, Freeman TB. A double-blind, randomized, controlled, multi-center clinical trial of the safety and efficacy of transplanted fetal porcine ventral mesencephalic cells versus imitation surgery in patients with Parkinson's disease. Mov Disord 2001;16:983-984.

92. Schraermeyer U, Heimann K. Current understanding on the role of retinal pigment epithelium and its pigmentation. Pigment Cell Res 1999;12(4):219-236.

93. Cherksey BD, Sapirstein VS, Geraci AL. Adrenal chromaffin cells on microcarriers exhibit enhanced long-term functional effects when implanted into the mammalian brain. Neuroscience 1996;75(2):657-664.

94. Watts RL, Raiser C, Stover NP, Cornfeldt M, Schweikert A, Allen R, et al. Stereotaxic intrastriatal implantation of retinal pigment epithelial cells attached to microcarriers in six advanced Parkinson disease (PD) patients: two year follow-up. Neurology 2003;60(5(suppl 1)):A164-165.

95. Snyder BJ, Olanow CW. Stem cell treatment for Parkinson's disease: an update for 2005. Curr Opin Neurol 2005;18(4):376-385.

96. Kirik D, Georgievska B, Bjorklund A. Localized striatal delivery of GDNF as a treatment for Parkinson disease. Nat Neurosci 2004;7(2):105-110.

97. Nutt JG, Burchiel KJ, Comella CL, Jankovic J, Lang AE, Laws ER, Jr., et al. Randomized, double-blind trial of glial cell line-derived neurotrophic factor (GDNF) in PD. Neurology 2003;60(1):69-73.

98. Gill SS, Patel NK, Hotton GR, O'Sullivan K, McCarter R, Bunnage M, et al. Direct brain infusion of glial cell line-derived neurotrophic factor in Parkinson disease. Nat Med 2003;9(5):589-595.

99. Patel NK, Bunnage M, Plaha P, Svendsen CN, Heywood P, Gill SS. Intraputamenal infusion of glial cell line-derived neurotrophic factor in PD: a two-year outcome study. Ann Neurol 2005;57(2):298-302.

100. Slevin JT, Gerhardt GA, Smith CD, Gash DM, Kryscio R, Young B. Improvement of bilateral motor functions in patients with Parkinson disease through the unilateral intraputaminal infusion of glial cell line-derived neurotrophic factor. J Neurosurg 2005;102(2):216-222.

101. Amgen press releases. http://www.amgen.com/media/media_pr_detail.jsp? 2004 and http://www.amgen.com/media/media_pr_detail.jsp? 2005.

102. Muramatsu S, Tsukada H, Nakano I, Ozawa K. Gene therapy for Parkinson's disease using recombinant adeno-associated viral vectors. Expert Opin Biol Ther 2005;5(5):663-671.

103. Chen Q, He Y, Yang K. Gene therapy for Parkinson's disease: progress and challenges. Curr Gene Ther 2005;5(1):71-80.

104. Feigin A, Kaplitt M, During M, et al. Gene therapy for Parkinson's disease with AAV-GAD: an open label, dose escalation, safety-tolerability trial. Mov Disord 2005;20:1236.

105. During MJ, Kaplitt MG, Stern MB, Eidelberg D. Subthalamic GAD gene transfer in Parkinson disease patients who are candidates for deep brain stimulation. Hum Gene Ther 2001;12(12):1589-1591.

106. Azzouz M, Martin-Rendon E, Barber RD, Mitrophanous KA, Carter EE, Rohll JB, et al. Multicistronic lentiviral vector-mediated striatal gene transfer of aromatic L-amino acid decarboxylase, tyrosine hydroxylase, and GTP cyclohydrolase I induces sustained transgene expression, dopamine production, and functional improvement in a rat model of Parkinson's disease. J Neurosci 2002;22(23):10302-10312.

107. Oxford Biomedica website: http://www.oxfordbiomedica.co.uk/prosavin.htm. Accessed November 26, 2005.

108. Avigen website: http://www.avigen.com/non_financial_release/2005/2005_Avigen_EarlyData_PDClinicalTrial_07180 5.htm. Accessed November 26, 2005.

109. Ceregene website http://www.ceregene.com/f-sci-park.html. Accessed November 26, 2005.

Chapter 11

1. Belluzzi JD, Domino EF, May JM, Bankiewicz KS, McAfee DA. N-0923, a selective dopamine D2 receptor agonist, is efficacious in rat and monkey models of Parkinson's disease. Mov Disord 1994;9:147-154.

2. Hutton JT, Metman LV, Chase TN, et al. Transdermal dopaminergic D(2) receptor agonist therapy in Parkinson's disease with N-0923 TDS: a double-blind, placebo-controlled study. Mov Disord 2001;16:459-463.

3. Metman LV, Gillespie M, Farmer C, et al. Continuous transdermal dopaminergic stimulation in advanced Parkinson's disease. Clin Neuropharmacol 2001;24:163-169.

4. Parkinson Study Group. A controlled trial of rotigotine monotherapy in early Parkinson's disease. Arch Neurol 2003;60:1721-1728.

5. Poewe W, Luessi F. Clinical studies with transdermal rotigotine in early Parkinson's disease. Neurology 2005;65(Suppl 1):S11-14.

6. Reynolds NA, Wellington K, Easthorpe SE. Rotigotine: in Parkinson's disease. CNS Drugs 2005;19:973-981.

7. Grondin R, Bedard PJ, Hadj Tahar A, Gregoire L, Mori A, Kase H. Antiparkinsonian effect of a new selective adenosine A2A receptor antagonist in MPTP-treated monkeys. Neurology 1999;52:1673-1677.

8. Hettinger BD, Lee A, Linden J, Rosin DL. Ultrastructural localization of adenosine A2A receptors suggests multiple cellular sites for modulation of GABAergic neurons in rat striatum. J Comp Neurol 2001;431:331-346.

9. Ochi M, Koga K, Kurokowa M, Kase H, Nakamura J, Kuwana Y. Systemic administration of adenosine A(2A) receptor antagonist reverses increased GABA release in the globus pallidus of unilateral 6-hydroxydopamine-lesioned rats: a microdialysis study. Neuroscience 2000;100:53-62.

10. Kanda T, Jackson MJ, Smith LA, et al. Adenosine A2A antagonist: a novel antiparkinsonian agent that does not provoke dyskinesia in parkinsonian monkeys. Ann Neurol 1998;43:507-513.

11. Kanda T, Jackson MJ, Smith LA, et al. Combined use of the adenosine A(2A) antagonist KW-6002 with L-DOPA or with selective D1 or D2 dopamine agonists increases antiparkinsonian activity but not dyskinesia in MPTP-treated monkeys. Exp Neurol 2000;162:321-327.

12. Hauser RA, Hubble JP, Truong DD, Group IU-S. Randomized trial of the adenosine A(2A) receptor antagonist istradefylline in advanced PD. Neurology 2003;61:297-303.

13. Bara-Jimenez W, Sherzai A, Dimitrova T, et al. Adenosine A(2A) receptor antagonist treatment of Parkinson's disease. Neurology 2003;61:293-296.

14. Goetz CG, Tanner CM, Klawans HL. Bupropion in Parkinson's disease. Neurology 1984;34:1092-1094.

15. Parkes JD, Tarsy D, Marsden CD, et al. Amphetamines in the treatment of Parkinson's disease. J Neurol Neurosurg Psychiatry 1975;38:232-237.

16. Frackiewicz EJ, Jhee SS, Shiovitz TM, et al. Brasofensine treatment for Parkinson's disease in combination with levodopa/carbidopa. Ann Pharmacother 2002;36:225-230.

17. Pearce RK, Smith LA, Jackson MJ, Banerji T, Scheel-Kruger J, Jenner P. The monoamine reuptake blocker brasofensine reverses akinesia without dyskinesia in MPTP-treated and levodopa-primed common marmosets. Mov Disord 2002;17:877-886.

18. Bara-Jimenez W, Dimitrova T, Sherzai A, Favit A, Mouradian MM, Chase TN. Effect of monoamine reuptake inhibitor NS 2330 in advanced Parkinson's disease. Mov Disord 2004;19:1183-1186.

19. Niznik HB, Fogel EF, Fassos FF, Seeman P. The dopamine transporter is absent in parkinsonian putamen and reduced in the caudate nucleus. J Neurochem 1991;56:192-198.

20. Bara-Jimenez W, Bibbiani F, Morris MJ, et al. Effects of serotonin 5-HT1A agonist in advanced Parkinson's disease. Mov Disord 2005;20:932-936.

21. Bibbiani F, Oh JD, Chase TN. Serotonin 5-HT1A agonist improves motor complications in rodent and primate parkinsonian models. Neurology 2001;57:1829-1834.

22. Henry B, Fox SH, Peggs D, Crossman AR, Brotchie JM. The alpha2-adrenergic receptor antagonist idazoxan reduces dyskinesia and enhances anti-parkinsonian actions of L-Dopa in the MPTP-lesioned primate model of Parkinson's disease. Mov Disord 1999;14:744-753.

23. Konitsiotis S, Blanchet PJ, Verhagen L, Lamers E, Chase TN. AMPA receptor blockade improves levodopa-induced dyskinesia in MPTP monkeys. Neurology 2000;54:1589-1595.

24. Manson AJ, Iakovidou E, Lees AJ. Idazoxan is ineffective for levodopa-induced dyskinesias in Parkinson's disease. Mov Disord 2000;15:336-337.

25. Rascol O, Arnulf I, Peyro-Saint Paul H, et al. Idazoxan, an alpha-2 antagonist, and L-DOPA-induced dyskinesias in patients with Parkinson's disease. Mov Disord 2001;16:708-713.

26. Freed CR, Greene PE, Breeze RE, et al. Transplantation of embryonic dopamine neurons for severe Parkinson's disease. N Engl J Med 2001;344:710-719.

27. Olanow CW, Goetz CG, Kordower JH, et al. A double-blind controlled trial of bilateral fetal nigral transplantation in Parkinson's disease. Ann Neurol 2003;54:403-414.

28. Snyder BJ, Olanow CW. Stem cell treatment for Parkinson's disease: an update for 2005. Curr Opin Neurol 2005;18:376-385.

29. Lindvall O, Kokaia Z, Martinez-Serrano A. Stem cell therapy for human neurodegenerative disorders - how to make it work. Nat Med 2004;10:542-550.

30. Ben-Hur T, Idelson M, Khaner H, et al. Transplantation of human embronic stem cell-derived neural progenitors improves behavioral deficit in Parkinsonian rats. Stem Cellls 2004;22:1246-1255.

31. Park CH, Minn YK, Lee JY, et al. In vitro and in vivo analyses of human embryonic stem cell-derived dopamine neurons. J Neurochem 2005;92:1265-1276.

32. Perrier AL, Tabar V, Barberi T, et al. Derivation of midbrain dopamine neurons from human embryonic stem cells. Proc Natl Acad Sci USA 2004;101:12543-12548.

33. Schulz TC, Noggle SA, Palmarini GM, et al. Differentiation of human embryonic stem cells to dopaminergic neurons in serum-free suspension culture. Stem Cells 2004;22:1218-1238.

34. Yan Y, Yang D, Zarnowska ED, et al. Directed differentiation of dopaminergic neuronal subtypes from human embryonic stem cells. Stem Cells 2005;23:781-790.

35. Zeng X, Cai J, Chen J, et al. Dopaminergic differentiation of human embryonic stem cells. Stem Cellls 2004;22:925-940.

36. Takagi Y, Takahashi J, Saiki H, et al. Dopaminergic neurons generated from monkey embryonic stem cells function in a Parkinson primate model. J Clin Invest 2005;115:102-109.

37. Jin G, Tan X, Tian M, et al. The controlled differentiation of human neural stem cells into TH-immunoreactive (ir) neurons in vitro. Neurosci Lett 2005;386:105-110.

38. Kishi Y, Takahashi J, Koyanagi M, et al. Estrogen promotes differentiation and survival of dopaminergic neurons derived from human neural stem cells. J Neurosci Res 2005;79:279-286.

39. Liste I, Garcia-Garcia E, Martinez-Serrano A. The generation of dopaminergic neurons by human neural stem cells is enhanced by Bcl-XL, both in vitro and in vivo. J Neurosci 2004;24:10786-10795.

40. Wang X, Lu Y, Zhang H, et al. Distinct effects of pre-differentiated versus intact fetal mesencephalon-derived human neural progenitor cells in alleviating rat model of Parkinson's disease. Int J Dev Neurosci 2004;22:175-183.

41. Yang M, Donaldson AE, Marshall CE, Shen J, Iacovitti L. Studies on the differentiation of dopaminergic traits in human neural progenitor cells in vitro and in vivo. Cell Transplant 2004;13:535-547.

42. Dezawa M, Kanno H, Hoshino M, et al. Specific induction of neuronal cells from bone marrow stromal cells and application for autologous transplantation. J Clin Invest 2004;113:1701-1710.

43. Höglinger GU, Rizk P, Muriel MP, et al. Dopamine depletion impairs precursor cell proliferation in Parkinson disease. Nat Neurosci 2004;7:726-735.

44. Bakay RA, Raiser CD, Stover NP, et al. Implantation of Spheramine in advanced Parkinson's disease (PD). Front Biosci 2004;9:592-602.

45. Wu SS, Frucht SJ. Treatment of Parkinson's disease: what's on the horizon? CNS Drugs 2005;19:723-743.

46. Kearns CM, Cass WA, Smoot K, Kryscio R, Gash DM. GDNF protection against 6-OHDA: time dependence and requirement for protein synthesis. J Neurosci 1997;17:7111-7118.

47. Kearns CM, Gash DM. GDNF protects nigral dopamine neurons against 6-hydroxydopamine in vivo. Brain Res 1995;672:104-111.

48. Tomac A, Lindqvist E, Lin LF, et al. Protection and repair of the nigrostriatal dopaminergic system by GDNF in vivo. Nature 1995;373:289-290.

49. Gash DM, Zhang Z, Ovadia A, et al. Functional recovery in parkinsonian monkeys treated with GDNF. Nature 1996;380:252-255.

50. Grondin R, Zhang Z, Yi A, et al. Chronic, controlled GDNF infusion promotes structural and functional recovery in advanced parkinsonian monkeys. Brain 2002;125:2191-2201.

51. Miyoshi Y, Zhang Z, Ovadia A, et al. Glial cell line-derived neurotrophic factor-levodopa interactions and reduction of side effects in parkinsonian monkeys. Ann Neurol 1997;42:208-214.

52. Nutt JG, Burchiel KJ, Comella CD, et al. Randomized, double-blind trial of glial cell line-derived neurotrophic factor (GDNF) in PD. Neurology 2003;60:69-73.

53. Kordower JH, Palfi S, Chen EY, et al. Clinicopathological findings following intraventricular glial-derived neurotrophic factor treatment in a patient with Parkinson's disease. Ann Neurol 1999;46:419-424.

54. Gill SS, Patel NK, Hotton GR, et al. Direct brain infusion of glial cell line-derived neurotrophic factor in Parkinson disease. Nat Med 2003;9:589-595.

55. Schapira AHV. Present and future drug treatment for Parkinson's disease. J Neurol Neurosurg Psychiatry 2005;76:1472-1478.

56. Kishima H, Poyot T, Bloch J, et al. Encapsulated GDNF-producing C2C12 cells for Parkinson's disease: a pre-clinical study in chronic MPTP-treated baboons. Neurobiol Dis 2004;16:428-439.

57. Sajadi A, Bauer TM, Thony B, Aebischer P. Long-term glial cell line-derived neurotrophic factor overexpression in the intact nigrostriatal system in rats leads to a decrease of dopamine and increase of tetrahydrobiopterine production. J Neurochem 2005;93:1482-1486.

58. Kordower JH, Emborg ME, Bloch J, et al. Neurodegeneration prevented by lentiviral vector delivery of GDNF in primate models of Parkinson's disease. Science 2000;290:767-773.

59. During MJ, Kaplitt MG, Stern MB, Eidelberg D. Subthalamic GAD gene transfer in Parkinson disease patients who are candidates for deep brain stimulation. Hum Gene Ther 2001;12:1589-1591.

60. Luo J, Kaplitt MG, Fitzsimons HL, et al. Subthalamic GAD gene therapy in a Parkinson's disease rat model. Science 2002;298:425-429.

61. Eberhardt O, Schulz JB. Gene therapy in Parkinson's disease. Cell Tissue Res 2004;318:243-260.

62. Vila M, Pzredborski S. Genetic clues to the pathogenesis of Parkinson's disease. Nat Med 2004;10 Suppl:S58-62.

63. Ravina BM, Fagan SC, Hart RG, et al. Neuroprotective agents for clinical trials in Parkinson's disease. Neurology 2003;60:1234-1240.

64. Group PS. Effects of tocopherol and deprenyl on the progression of disability in early Parkinson's disease. N Engl J Med 1993;328:176-183.

65. Olanow CW, Hauser RA, Gauger L, et al. The effects of deprenyl and levodopa on the progression of Parkinson's disease. Ann Neurol 1995;38:833-834.

66. Group PS. Impact of deprenyl and tocopherol treatment on Parkinson's disease in DATATOP patients requiring levodopa. Ann Neurol 1996;39:946-948.

67. Group PS. A controlled, randomized, delayed-start study of rasagiline in early Parkinson disease. Arch Neurol 2004;61:561-566.

68. Shults CW, Oakes D, Kieburtz K, et al. Effects of coenzyme Q10 in early Parkinson disease: evidence of slowing of the functional decline. Arch Neurol 2002;59:1541-1550.

69. Hartmann A, Hunot S, Michel PP, et al. Caspase-3: A vulnerability factor and final effector in apoptotic death of dopaminergic neurons in Parkinson's disease. Proc Natl Acad Sci USA 2000;97:2875-2880.

70. Klettner A, Herdegen T. FK506 and its analogs - therapeutic potential for neurological disorders. Curr Drug Target CNS Neurol Disord 2003;2:153-162.

71. Du Y, Ma Z, Lin S, et al. Minocycline prevents nigrostriatal dopaminergic neurodegeneration in the MPTP model of Parkinson's disease. Proc Natl Acad Sci USA 2001;98:14669-14674.

72. Parkinson Study Group. The safety and tolerability of a mixed lineage kinase inhibitor (CEP-1347) in PD. Neurology 2004;62:330-332.

73. Stocchi F, Olanow CW. Neuroprotection in Parkinson's disease: Clinical trials. Ann Neurol 2003;53:S87-S89.

74. Parkinson Study Group. Dopamine transporter brain imaging to assess the effects of pramipexole vs levodopa on Parkinson disease progression. JAMA 2002;287(13):1653-1661.

75. Whone AL, Watts RL, Stoessl AJ, et al. Slower progression of Parkinson's disease with ropinirole versus levodopa: The REAL-PET study. Ann Neurol 2003;54:93-101.

76. Oertel WH, Wolters E, Sampaio C, et al. Pergolide versus levodopa monotherapy in early Parkinson's disease patients: The PELMOPET study. Mov Disord, in press.

77. Fahn S. Does levodopa slow or hasten the rate of progression of Parkinson's disease? J Neurol 2005;252(Suppl 4):iv37-iv42.

ACKNOWLEDGEMENTS

Figure 1-1.   Reprinted with kind permission from Duvoisin RC, Sage J. Parkinson's Disease: A Guide for Patient and Family. 4th Edition. Lippincot-Raven, 1996.

Figure 1-2.   Reprinted with kind permission from Springer-Verlag, Braak et al. Cell Tissue Res. (2004); 318:121-134

Figure 1-3.   Reprinted with kind permission from Jankovic J, Tolosa E, Eds. Parkinson's Disease and Movement Disorders. Williams and Wilkins, 1993.

Figure 1-6.   Reprinted with kind permission from Calne DB. Parkinsonism: Physiology, Pharmacology and Treatment. Edward Arnold, 1970.

Figure 1-8.   Reprinted with kind permission from Calne DB. New England Journal of Medicine 1993;329:1022.

Figure 1-9.   Reprinted with kind permission from Calne DB. New England Journal of Medicine 1993;329:1023.

Figure 1-10. Reprinted with kind permission from Calne DB. New England Journal of Medicine 1993;329:1023.

Figure 2-2.   Reprinted with kind permission from Cedarbaum JM, Grancher ST. Neurologic Clinics 1992;10:544.

Table 4-1.   SIC Task Force appraisal of clinical diagnostic criteria for parkinsonian disorders Reprinted with kind permission of John Wiley & Sons, Inc., Litvan et al. Mov Disord. 2003 May;18(5):467-86.

Chapter 5   Patient Symptoms Questionnaire, Reprinted with kind permission from John Wiley & Sons, Inc.Movement Disorders Society, Mov Disord. 2005, Vol 20(6): 726-733

Chapter 5   Frequency of Wearing-Off, Reprinted with kind permission from John Wiley & Sons, Inc.,Movement Disorders Society, Mov Disord. 2005, M Stacy et al, Vol 20(6): 726-733.

Chapter 6   Jenner, P et al; Multiple small doses of levadopa plus entacapone produce continuous dopaminergic stimulation and reduce dyskinesia induction in MPTP treated drug naive primates Reprinted with kind permission of Movement Disord, Oct.2004;20(3).

Chapter 6   A controlled, randomized, delayed-start study of Rasigaline in early Parkinson's disease. Parkinson's Study Group. Reprinted with kind permission of Arch Neurol. 2004;61:561-566

Figure 6-1.   Reprinted with kind permission from Kaakkola S. Rinne UK, Gordin A. COMT Inhibition with Entacapone: a New Principle of Levodopa Extension. Koteva Oy, Tahitorni Oy; Finland 1996:13.

Figure 6-2.   Reprinted with kind permission from Kaakkola S. Rinne UK, Gordin A. COMT Inhibition with Entacapone: a New Principle of Levodopa Extension. Koteva Oy, Tahitorni Oy; Finland 1996:14.

Figure 6-3.   Reprinted with kind permission from Gordin A, Rinne UK. Rinne UK, Gordin A. COMT Inhibition with Entacapone: a New Principle of Levodopa Extension. Koteva Oy, Tahitorni Oy; Finland 1996:27.

Figure 6-7.   Reprinted with kind permission from Appel SH, Ed. Current Neurology 1992;12:130.

Figure 6-8.   Reprinted with kind permission from The Parkinson Study Group. New England Journal of Medicine 1993;328:178.
We would like to thank Kelly E. Lyons, PhD for suggestions and editorial comments

INDEX

NOTES

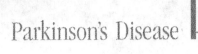